CONTENTS

CONTRIBUTORS

LOIS J. MARTYN

Associate Professor of Ophthalmology and Associate Professor in Pediatrics, Temple University School of Medicine, Philadelphia; Pediatric Ophthalmologist, St. Christopher's Hospital for Children, Philadelphia.

ANTHONY J. PILEGGI

Professor of Pediatrics, Temple University School of Medicine, Philadelphia; Director, Handicapped Children's Unit, St. Christopher's Hospital for Children, Philadelphia.

HENRY W. BAIRD

Professor of Pediatrics, Emeritus, Temple University School of Medicine, Philadelphia.

FOREWORD

The ophthalmological study of the child's eye allows an unique opportunity for documenting puzzling fundus changes. This technique demonstrates an intimate relationship between fundus changes and abnormalities which help us interpret difficult and often frustrating problems in the developmental and neurological disorders of children. The explosive developments in genetics, metabolic diseases, immunology, pathology, neonatology and other fields, including bio-engineering and sophisticated diagnostic techniques, have served to increase our awareness of subtle fundus and other ocular changes, revealing the clues which help us with the diagnosis.

I recall a fundus examination carried out more than 30 years ago on a child admitted for the ninth time for seizures of unknown origin. A large, white, elevated lesion in the mid-periphery of the fundus was diagnosed as tuberous sclerosis, allowing an understanding of this child's neurological disorder for the first time.

In addition to pointing out the pathological processes which can be observed, the authors of this monograph have also helped to make us aware of the wide range of fundal variations in both the normal- and delayed-developing posterior pole and retinal-pigment layer. The gradual sorting-out of this valuable collection of teaching material has required devotion and a great deal of time and patience. I congratulate the authors for making this valuable contribution to developmental pediatrics and child neurology, since it represents a significant step in the documentation of the causal-related changes observable in the abnormally developing child. It is hoped that their careful observations will stimulate other astute observers to build on this information and to improve our interpretation and understanding of this important aspect of pediatric neurology.

R. D. Harley, M.D., Ph.D.
Attending Surgeon,
Wills Eye Hospital,
Philadelpnia.
August 1984

PREFACE

The intent of the authors is to provide descriptions and brief discussions of optic fundus signs for use by students, residents in pediatrics and interested physicians. The book is written as a practical and useful guide for clinical evaluation. It is not an ophthalmological text, and detailed analyses are beyond its scope. We have included those conditons which we believe are of principal importance in caring for children with developmental and neurological disorders.

INTRODUCTION

Readily accessible for examination and subject to a wide range of developmental and pathological changes of both focal and systemic nature, the eyegrounds command special attention in the diagnosis of neurological disorders of childhood.

Of primary importance are the optic-nervehead signs of disease, such as papilledema, papillitis and optic atrophy, and a number of anomalies such as optic-nerve hypoplasia, aplasia and various colobomatous defects. Equally important are the retinal manifestations of neurological and systemic disease, including diffuse and focal chorioretinitis, the pigmentary retinal degenerations, a number of special maculopathies and the various retinal phakomata.

Essential to detection and proper interpretation of these signs are diligence and skill in the use of the ophthalmoscope, an appreciation of the range of variation in the appearance of the normal fundus, and an understanding of the ways in which pathological processes are manifested in the highly specialized tissues of the eye.

THE OPHTHALMOSCOPE

The standard, direct, hand-held ophthalmoscope consists basically of a source of light, devices to modify the projected beam of light, and a system of lenses to allow precise focusing of the image (Fig. 1).

Adequate light is important. Instruments that connect to house current *via* a transformer provide optimal light and are preferred by many clinicians. Most battery-operated ophthalmoscopes provide sufficient light for average clinical needs and are conveniently portable. However, the batteries must be kept well-charged, and the bulb should be replaced as often as necessary for optimal clarity. In both types, the intensity of the light can be controlled with a rheostat.

1

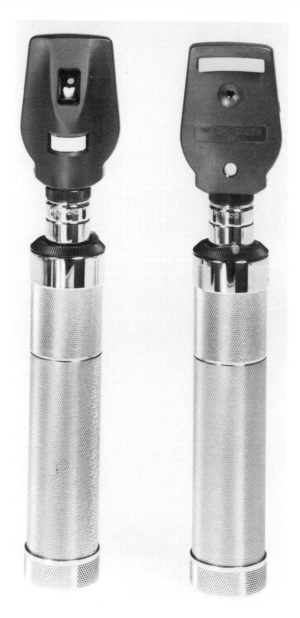

Figure 1.
The No. 11620 halogen co-axial ophthalmoscope from Welch Allyn. Photograph courtesy of Welch Allyn Inc., Skaneateles Falls, New York, USA.

The beam of light is modified by using the various apertures and accessories provided. In most instruments these include a small and a large round aperture, a vertical-slit aperture, a grid pattern and a red-free (green) filter. The small round aperture is used for viewing through a small pupil; the large round aperture for viewing through a large or dilated pupil. The vertical-slit aperture is intended for assessing the contour (convexity, concavity) of fundus lesions—elevated or depressed lesions produce bowing or step-like disruption of the slit-beam; flat lesions produce no distortion. The grid pattern can be used for gauging and recording the size of lesions or the caliber of vessels. The green lens or red-free light is used to help differentiate blood from pigment—blood (or old hemoglobin) appears dark black in red-free light, whereas melanin appears less black. The striations of the normal nerve-fiber pattern also are seen better in red-free light.

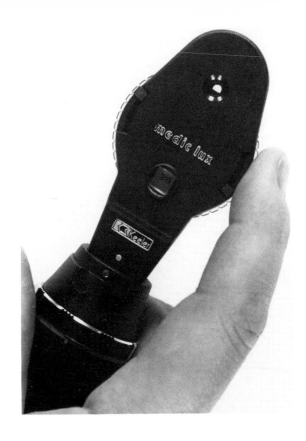

Figure 2.
Position of hand on
ophthalmoscope.

For focusing, the head of the direct ophthalmoscope contains a series of convex and concave lenses housed in a rotary disc. The convex or plus (+) lenses customarily are indicated by black numbers; the concave or minus (−) power lenses, by red numbers. The power of the lenses provided usually ranges from zero (plano) to plus and minus 15 or 20 diopters; in some instruments accessory lenses are included to provide as much as 40 diopters of lens power. To bring the image into focus, the examiner need only rotate the disc or 'dial in' sufficient power. The power or 'number' of the lens required will vary with the refractive state of both the examiner's eye and the patient's eye. If the examiner's refractive error is corrected with eye glasses, only the patient's refractive error need be neutralized or compensated for with the lenses. If the patient is very myopic and the examiner is having difficulty focusing on the retina, it may be helpful if the patient also puts on his glasses.

EXAMINATION TECHNIQUE

The instrument should be held securely, with the hand placed sufficiently far up on the barrel so that the forefinger can reach the rotary lens disc comfortably at all times (Fig. 2). This enables the examiner to change the dioptric power as needed throughout the examination.

The examiner uses his right hand and his right eye to examine the patient's right eye, his left hand and left eye to examine the patient's left eye.

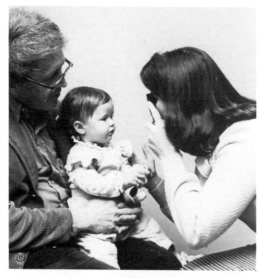

Figure 3.
Examination in the upright sitting position. Moving in slowly, one can often examine the optic fundus without upsetting or restraining child.

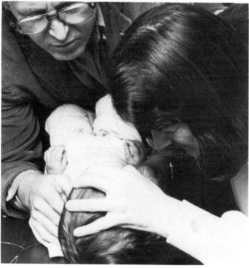

Figure 4.
Examination of infant lying on a flat surface. Child can be adequately and safely restrained by parent.

Both the examiner and patient must be positioned comfortably. With a little wooing, most children can be examined in the upright sitting position (Fig. 3). Infants often are better examined lying on a flat surface (Fig. 4) or cradled in the parent's arms. Examination also can be done well with the infant lying in the parent's lap with the baby's head resting on the knees and with his legs straddling the waist. By raising the baby's arms beside his head, the parent can restrain the infant securely but gently, while the examiner, sitting knee-to-knee with the parent, looks down over the top of the infant's head. It is also helpful if the infant sucks on a pacifier or bottle during the procedure.

Patience and a non-threatening approach are crucial to the successful examination of children. In the beginning it is important to touch the child as little as possible. In many cases, however, it becomes necessary to hold open the lids manually, or to restrain the child; this must be done gently, preferably by a member of the family or by an attendant

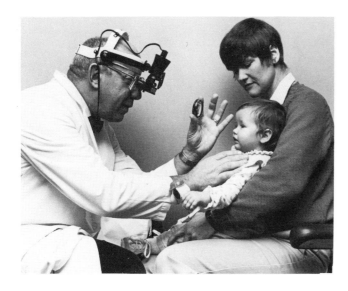

Figure 5.
Indirect
ophthalmoscopy.
Head lamp and
hand-held
condensing lens
are used to
visualize the optic
fundus.

experienced in handling apprehensive youngsters. The frightful practice of
strapping down a child is to be avoided. Talking to the child, humming or
playing soft music during the procedure may also help to calm the child.

Visualization of the inner eye can be augmented or facilitated by dilating
the pupils with mydriatic eyedrops.

Systematic ophthalmoscopy begins with examination of the outer eye
and assessment of the clarity of the 'red reflex' (the reddish-orange glow of
light reflected from the retina through the optical media). A high plus lens
(10 to 15 diopters) is used, with the instrument held 12 inches or so from
the eye. Any opacity such as a cataract or vitreous floater will cast a dark
shadow in the reflex. The reflex also may appear dark if the patient has a
high refractive error.

The examiner then progressively moves closer to the eye, simultaneously
reducing the plus power in the instrument by rotating the lens disc
counterclockwise (toward the minus side), gradually focusing more deeply
into the eye until the structures of the fundus come into clear view.

It is customary to examine the optic disc first; then each of the four
quadrants of the fundus, following the major vessel branches as far as
possible; and finally the macula. The disc is best seen by having the patient
look forward, while the examiner directs the light just nasal to the patient's
line of gaze. If one is 'lost' in the fundus, the disc can be located by tracing
the major vessels back to their origin. The more peripheral regions can be
brought into view by having the patient look as far as possible in the
direction of the intended examination, *i.e.* up and to the right for
examination of the right-upper temporal quadrant, down and to the left for
examination of the left-inferior temporal quadrant, and so forth. The
macula is brought into view by asking the patient to look directly into the
examiner's light. Examination of the far periphery requires full pupillary
dilatation and use of the indirect ophthalmoscope; skilful use of this
instrument requires considerable practice and is often left to the
ophthalmologist (Fig. 5).

THE NORMAL FUNDUS

The area of the fundus occupied by the ophthalmoscopically visible intra-ocular portion of the optic nerve is referred to as the disc. Anatomically it is referred to as the nervehead or papilla. It is composed of approximately 1 million nerve fibers converging from the retina to course through the optic nerve, chiasm and tracts to the lateral geniculate body. The structure is round to slightly oval, averaging 1.5 to 1.7mm, with its long axis vertical. It is somewhat nasal to the center of the globe. Often the nasal portion is fuller or more 'heaped up' than the temporal, owing to the greater number of nerve fibers coming into the nasal sector. The margins should be well defined. Normally the color is orange, ranging from yellow to pink. There is usually a paler central or paracentral depression referred to as the cup, occupying 30 per cent or less of the disc area. The major retinal vessels emerge from and converge into the cup area.

As the axons turn to course posteriorly into the nerve trunk, they traverse a sieve-like portion of the sclera, referred to as the cribiform plate. On ophthalmoscopic examination, grayish markings of this structure can often be visualized in the depth of the cup.

The central retinal artery emerging from the disc bifurcates into superior and inferior segments, each of which then divides into temporal and nasal branches that supply the four retinal quadrants. The vessels continue to branch further as they extend peripherally, curving gently in their course. On ophthalmoscopic examination the arteries (or, more correctly, arterioles) appear bright red with a lighter central stripe of reflected light.

The retinal veins converging into the disc follow a similar pattern of gently curving bifurcations, closely approximating those of the arterioles. Compared to the arterioles, the veins appear darker in color; they are also wider, having a ratio of 3:2 in diameter, and are somewhat more tortuous. Pulsation of the central retinal vein at the disc often can be seen as a normal finding.

The general background appearance of the fundus varies with the

6

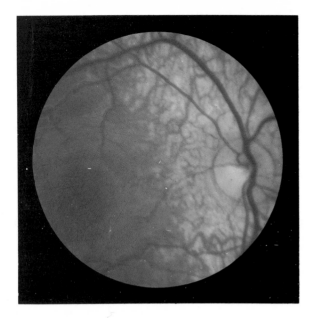

Figure A.
The normal fundus.
Landmarks are indicated in
the accompanying line
drawing.

Retinal artery

Macula

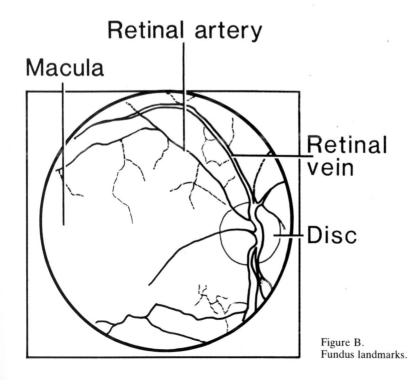

Retinal
vein

Disc

Figure B.
Fundus landmarks.

chorioretinal pigmentation. In deeply pigmented individuals the fundus has a uniform to somewhat mottled dark reddish, brick or slate color. In lightly pigmented individuals the fundus appears a paler yellowish-orange to light red, and the underlying choroidal vessels and sclera can be seen more clearly as interlacing broad ribbons of reddish-orange hue. The intervening areas of sclera visible to ophthalmoscopic examination appear pale yellow to white. Peripherally, the swirling orange pattern of large collecting veins, the vortex veins, may be seen.

The central area of the fundus, ophthalmoscopically and functionally, is the macula or foveal region. This is the highly specialized area of the retina that serves as the visual center of the eye, providing man's best visual acuity. The macula encompasses an area somewhat larger than the disc, approximately two disc diameters temporal to the disc. Owing to its highly specialized histological features, the macula is a slightly elevated mound with a shallow depression at its center. On ophthalmoscopic examination it generally appears somewhat darker than the rest of the fundus; in many individuals the mound is highlighted by soft light reflexes or demarcated by a narrow ring of light, and the central pit is marked by a bright focal light reflex or yellowish spot. The retinal vessels arch above and below the macula but do not extend directly into the macula, although a cilioretinal vessel coursing from the disc to the macula is present in some individuals.

With regard to general localization ophthalmoscopically, the area in and immediately around the macula is also referred to as the posterior pole. The area around the disc is called the peripapillary area; the intermediate zone is called the mid-periphery; and the region beyond is the far-periphery.

THE ABNORMAL FUNDUS

1 PAPILLEDEMA

Papilledema is characterized by various degrees of congestion, swelling and elevation of the nervehead; obliteration of the disc cup; edematous blurring of the disc margins; dilatation and tortuosity of the retinal veins; loss of spontaneous venous pulsation; and hemorrhages and exudates on and around the disc (Fig. 1a,b,c). There also may be concentric wrinkling of the retina, and extension of the edema, hemorrhages and exudates into the macular area.

Papilledema or 'choked disc' is of primary clinical importance as a cardinal sign of increased intracranial pressure. Swelling of the disc may occur, however, with a variety of other neurological processes and systemic diseases, and with a number of ocular and orbital conditions of diverse etiology (Fig. 1d).

The probable sequence of events producing papilledema in patients with increased intracranial pressure is as follows: elevation of intracranial subarachnoid cerebrospinal fluid pressure; elevation of cerebrospinal fluid pressure in the sheath of the optic nerve; elevation of tissue pressure in the optic nerve; stasis of axoplasmic flow; and swelling of the nerve fibers in the optic nervehead. The axon swelling then produces secondary vascular changes and the characteristic ophthalmoscopic signs of venous stasis.

In children, papilledema most often is associated with hydrocephalus, intracranial tumor, intracranial hemorrhage, or the cerebral edema of trauma, meningo-encephalitis or toxic encephalopathy. It should be noted, however, that in the infant or very young child with increased intracranial pressure, papilledema may not develop owing to distensibility of the skull and spreading of the cranial sutures.

As a rule, papilledema will resolve when the elevated intracranial pressure is alleviated, and the discs may return to a normal or nearly normal appearance within six to eight weeks. However, longstanding papilledema may lead to postpapilledema optic atrophy with attendant loss of vision and visual field.

To be differentiated from true papilledema are certain structural changes of the disc ('pseudopapilledema', 'pseudoneuritis', drusen and medullated fibers) that can mimic the appearance of disc swelling.

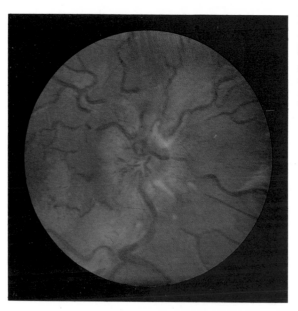

Figure 1a
Papilledema of increased intracranial pressure
There is hyperemia and swelling of nervehead, edema of retina, congestion and tortuosity of veins. Child had hydrocephalus.

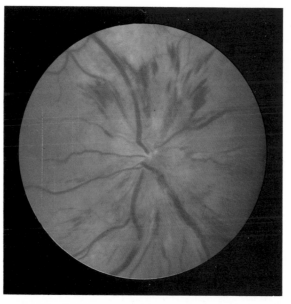

Figure 1b
Acute papilledema
In this patient with 'choked disc' of increased intracranial pressure, retinal hemorrhages are a prominent feature.

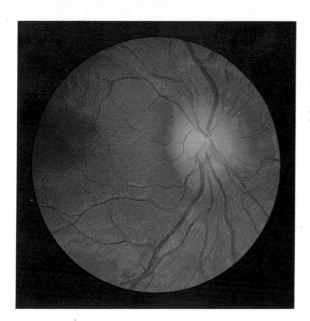

Figure 1c
Low-grade papilledema
Disc changes are minimal in this child with increased intracranial pressure secondary to an infiltrative tumor around aqueduct of Sylvius. Child presented with ataxia.

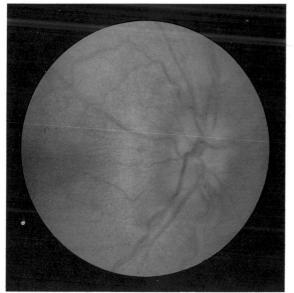

Figure 1d
Disc edema
Swelling of disc in this child was due to histiocytosis (Hand-Schueller-Christian disease).

2 OPTIC NEURITIS

Optic neuritis exists when there is active inflammation, degeneration or demyelinization of the optic nerve with attendant impairment of visual function. When the anterior portion of the nerve is involved, producing ophthalmoscopically visible disc changes, the term *papillitis* is applied; this is characterized by edema or swelling of the nervehead (Fig. 2a,b), often with hemorrhages and exudates. When there is nervehead and retinal involvement, the term optic *neuroretinitis* can be used. When the more posterior intra-orbital, intracanalicular or intracranial portion of the nerve is involved, producing no ophthalmoscopically visible nervehead changes, the term *retrobulbar neuritis* is applied. The condition may be unilateral or bilateral.

Optic neuritis generally is an acute process, accompanied by visual symptoms that commence abruptly and progress rapidly; the involved eye may become blind or nearly blind in a matter of hours or days, although often vision loss is less profound or in some cases even minimal. A variety of visual-field defects occur, of which central and centrocecal scotomas are most common. There is usually an attendant afferent pupillary defect. There may be pain on movement of the eye or on palpation of the eyes; discomfort or headache may precede or accompany the visual symptoms.

Optic neuritis rarely occurs in childhood as an isolated entity; it is usually a manifestation of more widespread neurological or systemic disease. It may occur with demyelinating disease such as disseminated sclerosis, Devic's neuromyelitis optica or Schilder's disease (adrenoleukodystrophy). It may also occur in association with infectious or para-infectious processes, often as a complication of bacterial or viral meningitis, or as a complication of encephalomyelitis, particularly following an exanthem, or even an immunization. Certain toxins should also be considered in the etiology of optic neuritis in children—for example, it may develop with lead poisoning, as a complication of long-term, high-dose chloramphenicol therapy, with certain antimetabolites, or as the result of the use of illicit drugs.

The prognosis in optic neuritis varies with the etiology. In many cases there is recovery, with improvement in vision; in other cases there is permanent visual impairment and some degree of optic atrophy.

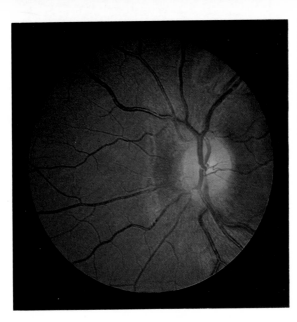

Figure 2a
Optic neuritis, acute
Note nerve-fiber layer edema. This 10-year-old patient presented with sudden loss of vision. She subsequently developed transverse myelitis, suggesting Devic's neuromyelitis optica.

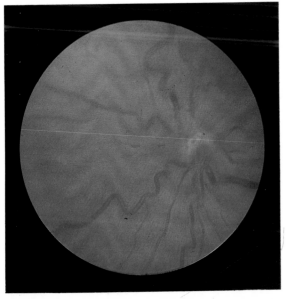

Figure 2b
Acute papillitis
This child developed acute optic neuritis consequent to long-term high-dose chloramphenicol treatment for cystic fibrosis. There is marked swelling of disc.

3 OPTIC ATROPHY

The term optic atrophy denotes degeneration of optic-nerve fibers with attendant impairment of function. The ophthalmoscopic signs are pallor and decreased vascularity of the disc, and loss of nervehead tissue, sometimes with enlargement of the optic cup (Fig. 3a,b,c,d). Clinical signs of impaired function vary with the nature and site of the primary lesion or disease process, and with the extent and severity of the damage; there may be localized visual-field defects, reduction or loss of central visual acuity, and signs of afferent (conduction) pupillary dysfunction.

Optic atrophy may result from disease within the eye or from disease affecting the intra-orbital, intracanalicular or intracranial portion of the anterior visual pathways. The causes are protean, including inflammatory processes, degenerative disorders, neoplastic disease, vascular disorders, trauma and toxic insults. Delineation of the etiology often requires extensive investigation, including neuroradiological, metabolic and genetic studies. However, the following generalizations may be of some practical clinical value in assessing children with optic atrophy.

Many children with optic atrophy have a readily identifiable, reasonable explanation for the atrophy. The problem often is long-standing and the course relatively stable. In this group are children with a well-documented past history of hypoxia or meningo-encephalitis and those with hydrocephalus, micrencephaly or craniosynostosis, or previous cranial trauma. There often is attendant developmental delay, a motor handicap, or seizure disorder. These children present little problem with regard to diagnosis, although documented progressive changes in the disc would warrant further investigation.

The previously normal child who develops progressive optic atrophy presents an entirely different diagnostic problem, and requires aggressive investigation for progressive neurological or systemic disease, intra-orbital or intracranial tumor. Craniopharyngioma, optic glioma and hydrocephalus are particularly frequent causes. A number of heredodegenerative optic atrophies that present in childhood also must be considered; diagnosis is based on careful family study and the clinical profile. In addition, glaucoma (increased intra-ocular pressure) must be ruled out in children with optic atrophy, particularly when there is enlargement or excavation of the optic cup.

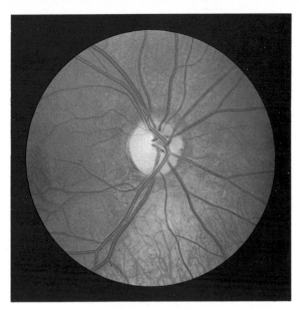

Figure 3a
Optic atrophy
This is the classical picture
of advanced optic atrophy.
Note pallor and decreased
vascularity of disc, and loss
of nervehead substance.

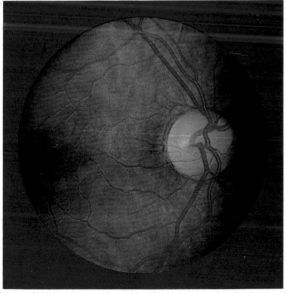

Figure 3b
Moderate optic atrophy
There is mild generalized
pallor of disc in this five
year-old child with
craniopharyngioma.

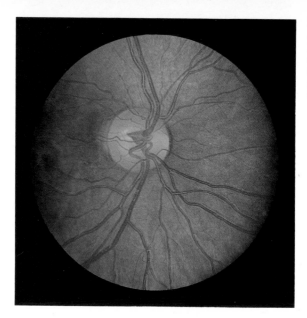

Figure 3c
Sector optic atrophy
In this child sector atrophy can be detected in temporal and nasal portions of disc as an early sign of brain tumor (craniopharyngioma).

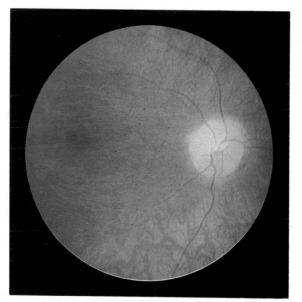

Figure 3d
Optic atrophy
Optic atrophy in this child is secondary to diffuse progressive nervous-system degeneration (lipofuscinosis). Note arteriolar attenuation.

A large or enlarged optic cup may occur as a normal developmental variant or as the result of disease.

In the absence of disease, the developmentally large cup, though broad and deep, tends to be relatively round or only slightly oval, and is surrounded by a rim of healthy nervehead tissue (Fig. 4a). In addition, within the spectrum of normal variation, the cup is usually equal or nearly equal in the two eyes. Genetic determination is a factor in cup size, and examination of other family members may be helpful in differential diagnosis.

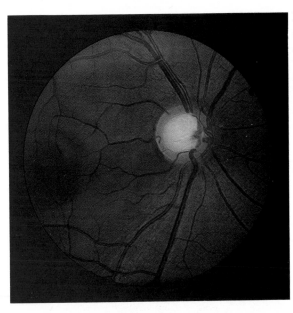

Figure 4a
Large disc cup
Vision and intra-ocular pressure were normal in this 10-year old boy with symmetrically large deep optic cups. Note rim of normal, pink nervehead tissue.

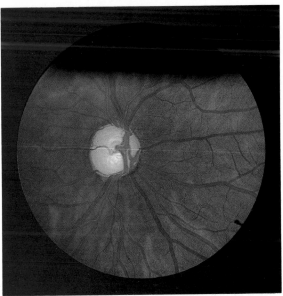

Figure 4b
Glaucomatous cupping
In this eight-year-old boy cup is enlarged and excavated, with pallor and atrophy of neuroretinal rim. Intra-ocular pressure was elevated abnormally and vision had been reduced to light perception. Fellow eye was normal.

To be differentiated from normal developmental variants are anomalies of the disc—colobomatous defects of the nervehead and optic-nerve hypoplasia, that may be characterized by the appearance of excavation.

Pathological enlargement and excavation of the cup, commonly referred to as 'cupping', is associated with glaucoma (Fig. 4b). In glaucoma the cup tends to show vertically oval or irregular enlargement, with pallor and atrophy of the neuroretinal rim, sometimes with 'notching' of the superior and inferior pole. The vessels also tend to become displaced nasally. In addition, significant difference between the cups of the two eyes is particularly suggestive of glaucoma. In infants and young children, other major signs of glaucoma are clouding (edema) of the cornea, photophobia and tearing, and progressive enlargement of the eye and cornea, referred to as buphthalmos. Ultimately there may be loss of vision.

In optic atrophy of other etiologies there may be some enlargement of the cup, but usually not the characteristic excavation and notching that occurs with the increased intra-ocular pressure of glaucoma.

OPTIC-NERVE PITS

Optic-nerve pits or 'holes' are considered to be minimal colobomatous defects. They appear as small round, oval, or slit-like craters or depressions, usually situated in the temporal portion of the disc (Fig. 5). There is often a diaphanous veil of grayish tissue filling-in or covering the defect. Optic-nerve pits may be associated with serous retinal detachment, and with vision and field defects that must be differentiated from those of progressive neurological disease.

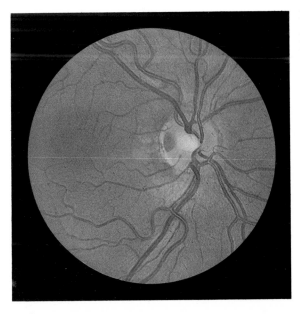

Figure 5
Optic pit
Note grayish oval defect in temporal portion of nervehead.

Optic-nerve hypoplasia is a developmental defect characterized by deficiency of optic-nerve fibers. It has been attributed to primary failure in the differentiation of retinal ganglion cells or their axons. However, it may result from prenatal degeneration of the ganglion-cell axons.

The defect may be unilateral or bilateral, mild to severe, with a broad spectrum of ophthalmoscopic findings and attendant clinical manifestations.

In typical cases the nervehead is small, occupying only a portion of the usual disc area, and leaving a pale or pigmented crescent or halo between the margin of the existent nervehead tissue and the margin of the pigmented retinal epithelium and choroid. This gives rise to the so-called 'double-ring' sign of optic-nerve hypoplasia. The nervehead tissue present usually is pale, although sometimes relatively pink. Paucity of tissue, however, is the principal diagnostic criterion (Fig. 6a,b,c,d). The major vessels generally are normal, although in some cases they are tortuous or attenuated. There is attendant hypoplasia of the macula; it appears flat, lacking its normal contours and light reflexes.

The attendant vision impairments range in severity from localized visual-field defects or minimal reduction in acuity to blindness of one or both eyes. In association with vision impairment there is often strabismus or nystagmus; abnormal eye movements or malalignment may be the presenting sign.

Optic-nerve hypoplasia may occur as an isolated defect in otherwise normal individuals, or in association with other abnormalities including anencephaly, hydranencephaly, hydrocephalus and meningo-encephalocele.

Hypoplasia of the optic nerves, chiasm and optic tracts may occur in association with absence of the septum pellucidum with a large chiasmatic cistern, an anomaly referred to as septo-optic dysplasia or deMorsier syndrome. There may be associated hypothalamic involvement, with endocrine disorders ranging from panhypopituitarism to isolated deficiency of growth hormone, hypothyroidism, diabetes insipidus or diabetes mellitus.

The exact cause of optic-nerve hypoplasia is unknown. It does not appear to be familial, although it has occurred in siblings. There is no chromosomal defect regularly associated with it. It may occur with somewhat increased frequency in infants of diabetic mothers.

To be differentiated from optic-nerve hypoplasia is optic-nerve aplasia. This is a rare anomaly in which there is absence of the optic nerve and of the retinal vessels. This condition presumably results from failure of the paraxial mesoderm to grow into the optic stalk before closure of the fetal fissure. Optic-nerve aplasia rarely occurs in otherwise normal individuals. It is usually associated with malformation of the globes or brain.

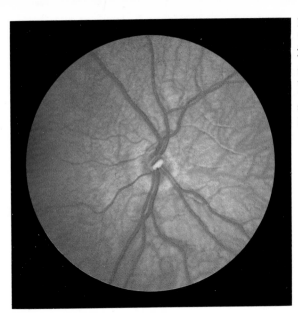

Figure 6a
Optic-nerve hypoplasia of severe degree
There is minimal nervehead tissue around central retinal vessels. Note pale halo or 'double-ring sign' encircling small donut of pink papillary tissue.

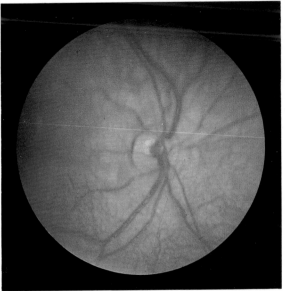

Figure 6b
Optic-nerve hypoplasia of moderate degree
Disc is just slightly smaller than normal, relatively pink, but flat and slightly deficient in nervehead tissue.

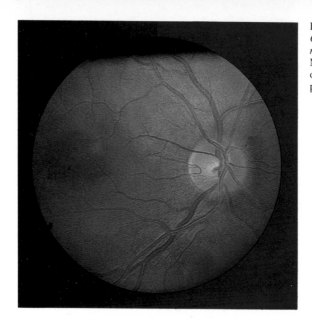

Figure 6c
Optic-nerve hypoplasia of minimal degree
Nervehead is small. There is only slight indication of a partial peripapillary ring.

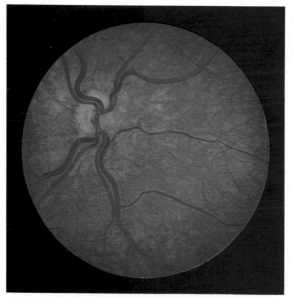

Figure 6d
Typical double-ring sign of optic-nerve hypoplasia
Double-ring sign in this infant is prominent.

TILTED DISC

Tilted optic disc is an anomaly in which one portion of the disc is displaced forward and appears elevated or 'full'; the opposite sector of the disc appears flat or recessed and often is bordered with a crescent or conus (Fig. 7). The disc may be tilted in any direction. The condition usually is bilateral. This anomaly is thought to be related to malclosure of the embryonic fissure. In conjunction with tilted disc there may be myopia and astigmatism, and vision and visual-field defects. The field defects often are bitemporal or altitudinal, and must be differentiated from those of acquired or progressive disease. In addition, the appearance of a tilted disc may mimic that of papilledema, as the margin of the elevated segment of the disc may appear 'blurred' on ophthalmoscopic examination.

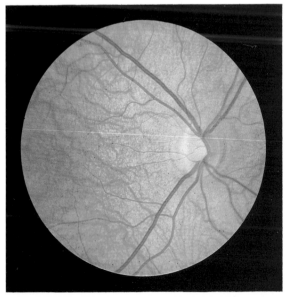

Figure 7
Tilted disc
Disc appears to be 'facing' macula; nasal portion of nervehead is prominent and displaced forward; the temporal portion of nervehead appears recessed and foreshortened; vessels appear to emerge from beneath temporal rim; and there is a pale crescent along temporal margin of disc.

Optic-disc drusen are globular, acellular bodies composed of concentric lamellae of hyalin material. They may be buried within the optic nervehead, producing smooth or irregular elevation of the disc that can be confused with papilledema (Fig. 8). Alternatively, the drusen may be partially or completely exposed, appearing as refractile bodies resembling tapioca pearls at the surface of the disc. The more superficial disc drusen often can be made to glow when transilluminated with oblique light. Fluorescein angiography, ultrasonography and computed axial tomography of the optic nerve also are useful in documenting the presence of intrapapillary drusen.

In some instances disc drusen are associated with nerve-fiber bundle or sector visual-field defects, enlargement of the blind spot, decreased visual acuity, and even with small spontaneous nerve fiber-layer hemorrhages adjacent to the disc.

The etiology of optic-disc drusen is unclear. They may occur as an autosomal dominant condition; examination of other family members may be helpful in making the diagnosis. Giant drusen of the disc have been associated with tuberous sclerosis of Bourneville.

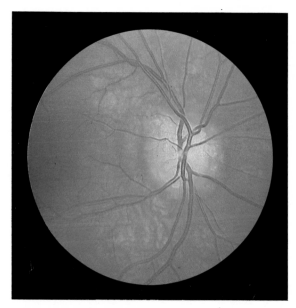

Figure 8
Optic-disc drusen
Note nodular elevation of nervehead and irregularity of disc margins due to hyalin bodies. Child was referred for evaluation of suspected papilledema; the clinical picture is that of pseudopapilledema.

PERSISTENT BERGMEISTER PAPILLA— EPIPAPILLARY MEMBRANE

Persistence of Bergmeister's papilla, often taking the form of an epipapillary membrane or glial tuft protruding from the disc, is a common developmental remnant.

Embryologically, as nerve fibers grow into the primitive epithelial papilla to form the optic nerve, a nidus of neuro-ectodermal cells becomes sequestered from the rest of the inner layer of the optic cup. At about the end of the fourth gestational month these cells multiply and form a glial sheath that extends around the hyaloid artery. During the seventh

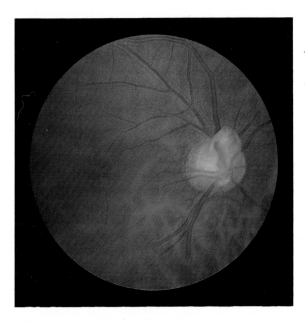

Figure 9a
Persistent Bergmeister papilla
Incomplete regression of Bergmeister's papilla in this child has left translucent tissue over disc with a cyst-like structure protruding into vitreous.

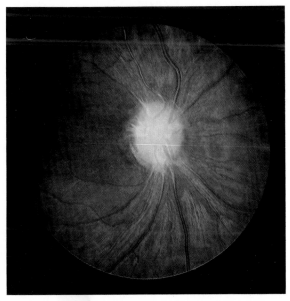

Figure 9b
Glial papillary veil
Persistent glial tissue over disc, as shown in this otherwise normal child, should not be confused with papilledema or papillitis. This is a developmental variant.

gestational month this tissue begins to atrophy. Incomplete regression may leave varying amounts of glial tissue. Ophthalmoscopically the appearance ranges from barely detectable glial tufts to conspicuous whitish veils over the disc, or globular or finger-like structures protruding into the vitreous (Fig. 9a,b). As a rule these developmental remnants do not affect visual function. These common developmental variants generally are easily recognized and should not be confused with inflammatory, hamartomatous or neoplastic conditions. The veils also must be differentiated from the disc changes of papilledema or papillitis.

PERSISTENT HYPERPLASTIC PRIMARY VITREOUS (PHPV)

Remnants of the vascular and fibrous elements of the primary vitreous may persist to varying degrees anywhere from the disc to the posterior surface of the lens, and in some individuals there is associated fibroblastic hyperplasia. This condition in its various forms is referred to as persistent hyperplastic primary vitreous or PHPV (Fig. 10a,b).

In full-blown or classical PHPV there is a retrolental mass or opacity, giving rise to a white reflex in the pupil. There is often prominence of the ciliary processes. The affected eye usually is microphthalmic or somewhat

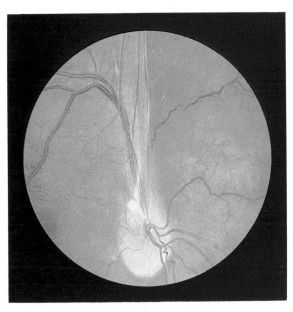

Figure 10a
Persistent hyperplastic primary vitreous
There is glial tissue extending superiorly from disc with associated traction on retina. Child subsequently developed a vitreous hemorrhage.

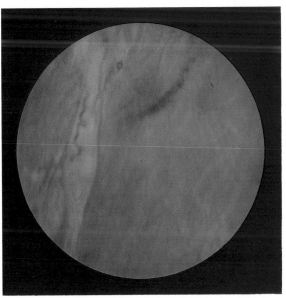

Figure 10b
PHPV
Note tube-like structure traversed by vessels lying anterior to retina. This is related to persistence of primary vitreous and hyaloid system.

smaller than normal. Associated complications include cataract, glaucoma, intra-ocular hemorrhage, retinal traction and detachment.

Lesser degrees of PHPV may be characterized by small remnants on the back surface of the lens. In other cases there is primarily involvement of the disc and retina. The ophthalmoscopic picture is often that of glial tissue over the disc. Fibroglial proliferation in the region of the disc may produce traction on the retina, leading to retinal fold or detachment.

In most cases PHPV is unilateral. Other ocular defects and systemic anomalies have been noted in some cases.

An unusual disc anomaly sometimes associated with PHPV, or possibly related developmentally to the whole spectrum of PHPV, is the so-called 'morning glory' disc anomaly. It may occur in association with other developmental defects including cleft palate, absence of the corpus callosum, sphenoidal encephalocele and renal abnormalities.

MYELINATED NERVE FIBERS

Whereas myelination of the optic-nerve fibers normally terminates at the level of the lamina cribosa, in some individuals myelination continues anterior to the lamina cribosa, resulting in ectopic medullation of the fibers of the optic nervehead and of the retina. On ophthalmoscopic examination, this area appears as a white or grayish-white patch, having a striated or feathered edge (Fig. 11).

There may be a relative or absolute visual-field defect corresponding to the area of ectopic medullation, or associated refractive error (myopia), strabismus or ambylopia. Otherwise, the eye usually is normal, although a variety of defects, including coloboma and cranial anomalies, has been reported in association with ectopic medullation. Ectopic medullation is also said to occur with increased frequency in von Recklinghausen neurofibromatosis.

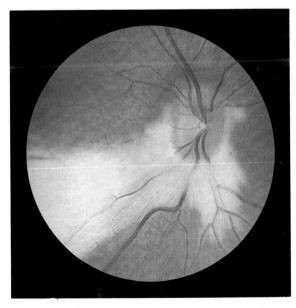

Figure 11
Medullated nerve fibers
This 'painted-on' brush-stroke appearance is characteristic of ectopic myelination of retinal-nerve fibers.

12 PERIPAPILLARY CRESCENTS

When the retinal-pigment epithelium or choroid fails to abut the margin of the disc, a peripapillary crescent may be seen (Fig. 12). This is a common developmental anomaly; congenital crescents are located most frequently on the temporal side of the disc and are often demarcated by extra pigmentation. They also occur in some individuals with myopia.

Developmental crescents usually are well defined and should not be confused with inflammatory or degenerative conditions.

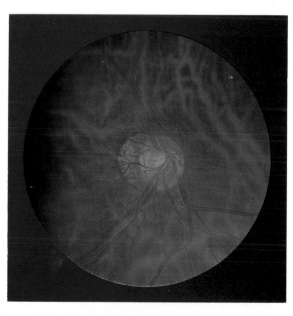

Figure 12
Peripapillary crescent
In this darkly pigmented child retinal-pigment epithelium falls short of disc margin, leaving a peripapillary choroidal crescent.

3 COLOBOMATA

The term coloboma describes a defect (gap, notch, fissure, hole) in which tissue or a portion of a tissue or structure is lacking. The principal types of ocular colobomata are (1) chorioretinal or fundus coloboma, with or without iris, ciliary body or optic-nerve involvement; and (2) isolated optic-nerve coloboma.

The typical fundus coloboma arises from malclosure of the embryonic fissure; this results in a defect in the retina, retinal-pigment epithelium and choroid, baring the sclera. The usual appearance is that of a well-circumscribed, wedge-shaped white area (exposed sclera) extending inferonasally below the disc, sometimes involving or engulfing the disc (Fig. 13a,b). In extreme cases there is cyst formation or ectasia in the area of the cleft. Alternatively, chorioretinal colobomata may be small focal defects appearing as single or multiple punched-out lesions or pigmentation in the line of the embryonic fissure (Fig. 13c,d). The defect may be unilateral or bilateral.

As a rule, there is a visual-field defect corresponding to the area of the chorioretinal defect. Visual acuity may be impaired, particularly if the optic nerve or macula is involved. The visual-field defects of this congenital anomaly must be differentiated from those of progressive disease.

Chorioretinal colobomata may occur unassociated with other abnormalities, as a sporadic defect or inherited as a dominant or recessive condition, or in association with other anomalies such as microphthalmia, cyclopia or anencephaly. They may occur in the syndromes of Patau (trisomy 13) or Edward (trisomy 18), with significant CNS abnormalties.

Isolated coloboma of the optic nerve, without the typical chorioretinal defect, may occur as a rare anomaly. In this condition the disc appears larger than normal, there is excavation and distortion of the disc, sometimes with a glial veil over the crater, and the blood vessels appear to traverse the border of the defect. There may be associated impairment of vision or field, but this is variable. This anomaly may be associated with trans-sphenoidal encephalocele, as well as with other system anomalies such as cardiac defects and a number of ocular abnormalities including posterior embryotoxon and posterior lenticonus. It may be familial.

A disc anomaly that may be related to coloboma of the optic disc is the 'morning glory' disc anomaly. In this condition the disc appears large with a funnel-shaped excavation and an annulus of elevated peripapillary tissue, sometimes pigmented. In some cases vision is subnormal. A variety of developmental abnormalities, including cleft lip and palate, agenesis of the corpus callosum and sphenoidal encephalocele, have been reported in association with the disc anomaly.

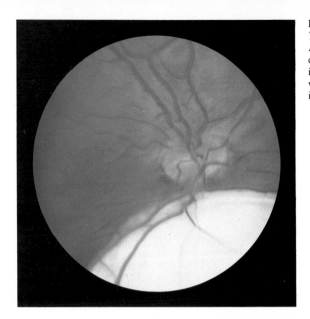

Figure 13a
Typical fundus coloboma
A well-demarcated
chorioretinal defect extends
inferonasally below disc. A
wedge-shaped area of sclera
is exposed.

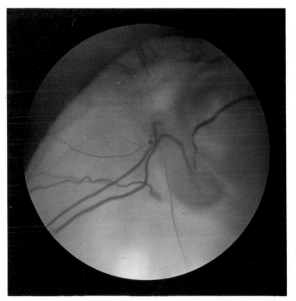

Figure 13b
Coloboma involving disc
This fundus coloboma
extends proximally,
engulfing disc. There is
marked distortion of disc
and vessels, and sclera is
ectatic.

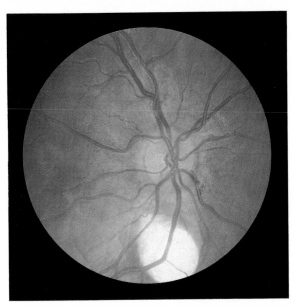

Figure 13c
*Focal chorioretinal
coloboma*
There is a discrete defect
inferior to disc; retinal
vessels traverse exposed
sclera.

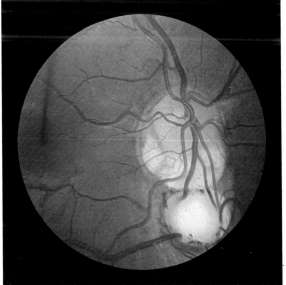

Figure 13d
*Fundus coloboma involving
disc*
In this child malclosure of
the embryonic fissure has
resulted in array of
contiguous defects. Note (1)
crescent-shaped defect
involving lower pole of disc;
(2) adjacent cavernous or
cyst-like defect with vessels
'climbing' rim; and (3)
sector of hypopigmentation
around defects and disc.

In clinical practice the term chorioretinitis is used in a broad sense to describe a variety of inflammatory changes of the choroid and retina. Pathologically, inflammation may arise primarily in the retina or in the choroid; the inflammation may be confined to these tissues, or the fundus changes may be just one facet of more extensive ocular inflammation.*

The causes are protean, and include both infectious and non-infectious processes. The clinical signs vary somewhat with the etiology, but certain generalizations can be made. As a rule, the acute phase is marked by cellular reaction with varying degrees of edema, exudation and hemorrhage; the involved areas of the fundus may appear hazy, gray or yellowish, there may be vascular sheathing, and the vitreous may appear cloudy owing to out-pouring of inflammatory cells (Fig. 14a,b). The process often results in necrosis and destruction of choroidal and retinal tissue, with dispersion and aggregation of pigment. In many cases the end result is permanent chorioretinal scarring—depending on the etiology and extent of the process, the ophthalmoscopic signs may vary from pigmentary mottling to discrete focal areas of chorioretinal atrophy appearing as white patches of exposed sclera, often well demarcated by dense clumps of pigmentation (Fig. 14c,d). There also may be gliotic veils or dense fibrotic membranes, retinal folds or detachment (Fig. 14e).

Whereas any number of infectious and non-infectious disease processes may be associated with chorioretinitis, those of special interest in pediatric practice are toxoplasmosis, cytomegalovirus disease and herpes virus infection, rubella, syphilis, tuberculosis and sarcoidosis, and toxocariasis.

The retinochoroiditis of congenital toxoplasmosis is usually characterized by focal atrophic and pigmented scars (Fig. 14f); large destructive lesions of the macular region are common. Rarely are there signs of active retinochoroiditis at birth. Active recurrences of the retinochoroiditis of toxoplasmosis may occur at any time in life, often resulting in satellite lesions adjacent to old scars. Detection of fundus lesions suggesting toxoplasmosis can be of diagnostic importance in the evaluation of an infant with signs of congenital infection syndrome, or in a child with developmental delay, retardation, microcephaly, intracranial calcifications or a seizure disorder.

Congenital cytomegalovirus infection and *Herpes simplex* infection acquired at birth may be seen as active chorioretinal inflammation in the infant, frequently accompanying signs of systemic infection or encephalitis. Vitreous haze, retinal edema and hemorrhages are common in the active phase; varying degrees of chorioretinal atrophy and pigmentation may follow. The chorioretinitis of *Herpes simplex* and cytomegalovirus may also

---

*It is common to classify ocular inflammation on the basis of the parts of the eye affected. Thus, inflammation of any part of the uveal tract generally can be referred to as uveitis, or more specifically as iritis, cyclitis, or choroiditis; it can be described as anterior or posterior uveitis depending on which segment is predominantly affected, or as panuveitis if all segments are involved. In many cases of uveitis there is inflammatory involvement of the contiguous retina, and the descriptive term chorioretinitis is applied. Similarly, inflammation arising in the retina may involve the underlying choroid; some prefer the term retinochoroiditis to make this distinction. Inflammation can be confined to the retina, and may be referred to as retinitis or as retinal vasculitis.

Visual symptoms vary considerably with the etiology and severity of the inflammatory process.

be seen as later-onset acquired disease, particularly as opportunistic infection in children on immunosuppressive therapy (Fig. 14g).

The fundus changes of congenital rubella are those of a pigmentary retinopathy, commonly of the 'salt and pepper' type, and are best described separately (see p. 41).

Congenital syphilis is relatively rare today, but may be seen as active choroiditis in the infant, or as secondary pigmentary changes detected later.

In sarcoidosis, retinal vascular signs are prominent. Perivenous infiltrates are common. There may be denser white inflammatory accumulations along retinal vessels resembling candle-wax drippings (Fig. 14h,i). Retinal edema, scattered exudates and hemorrhages also are common findings.

Tuberculous lesions in children are rarely seen, but miliary lesions of the choroid may develop in some children with generalized miliary tuberculosis and tuberculous meningitis. Clinically, these appear as ill-defined pale yellow, rounded lesions.

The fundus lesion of *Toxocara canis* usually is a unilateral focal lesion. On ophthalmoscopic examination it appears as an elevated white or grayish mass (Fig. 14j), most commonly located posteriorly in the macular region but sometimes situated peripherally along the ora serata, often with a transvitreal band. The vitreous may be hazy. The mass may give rise to the so-called cat's eye reflex or leukocoria—an opalescent reflection or white spot seen through the pupil.

As indicated by these few examples, in many patients with fundus signs of inflammatory disease, the clinical picture gives a clue to the etiology. It should be noted, however, that in many cases the signs are non-specific, and frequently the etiological agent cannot be identified, even after extensive investigation.

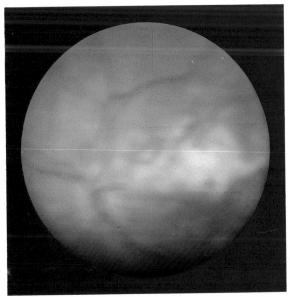

Figure 14a
Acute chorioretinitis
Acute inflammatory process is marked by exudation and edema, with haziness of fundus detail.

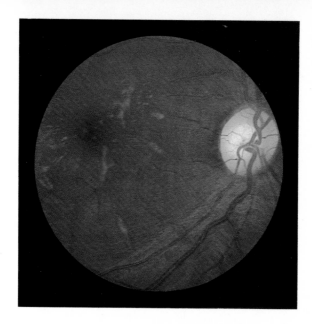

Figure 14b
Acute retinitis
Note retinal edema and exudation. Child presented with acute encephalitis, thought to be viral.

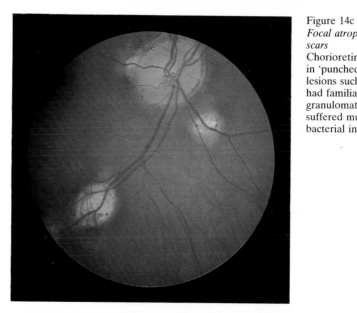

Figure 14c
Focal atrophic chorioretinal scars
Chorioretinitis often results in 'punched-out' atrophic lesions such as these. Child had familial chronic granulomatous disease and suffered multiple bouts of bacterial infection.

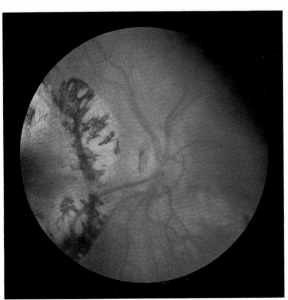

Figure 14d
Typical chorioretinal scar
Large areas of chorioretinal atrophy demarcated by dense pigmentation are common end-result of destructive inflammatory process in many patients with chorioretinitis.

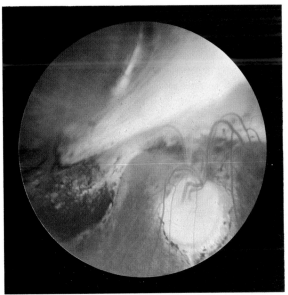

Figure 14e
Extensive chorioretinal scarring
Note chorioretinal atrophy, dense pigmentation, gliosis, retinal-vessel distortion and optic atrophy, all postinflammatory.

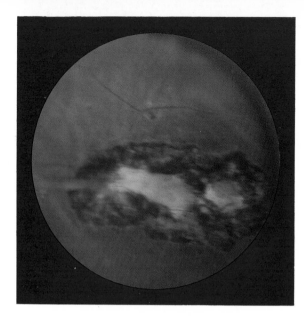

Figure 14f
Toxoplasmic chorioretinal scar
Large atrophic and pigmented scar near macula in this young girl with toxoplasmosis is typical of destructive lesions that so often occur in this disease. Satellite lesions are common.

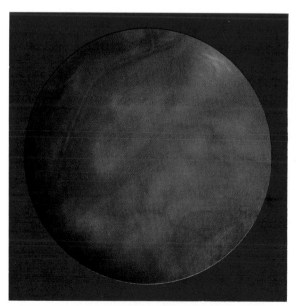

Figure 14g
Cytomegalovirus chorioretinitis
There is widespread edema and exudation of acute inflammation. This black child was on immunosuppressive drugs following kidney transplant.

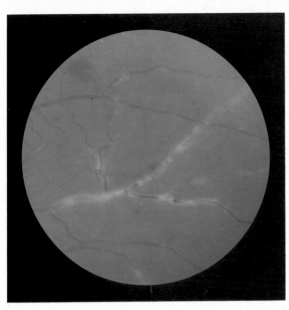

Figure 14h
Sarcoid retinitis
Perivascular exudates, likened to candle-wax drippings, retinal edema and scattered retinal hemorrhages are prominent features in this young boy with sarcoidosis.

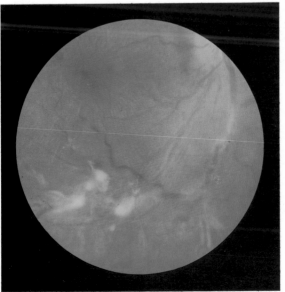

Figure 14i
Sarcoid retinitis
Note haze of widespread edema, perivascular exudates, and retinal hemorrhages.

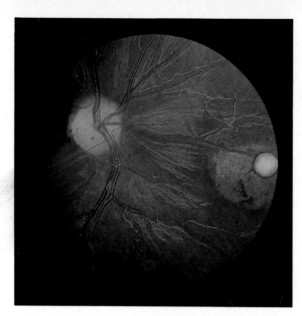

Figure 14j
Toxocara lesion
In this child with
toxocariasis, there is
elevated cystic lesion
contiguous to a retinal
vessel, in association with
background pigmentary
changes of fundus.

5 'SALT AND PEPPER' RETINOPATHY

'Salt and pepper' retinopathy is not a specific entity but rather a descriptive term applied to the retinal pigmentary changes seen in a number of diseases. The ophthalmoscopic picture is that of fine to coarse pigment stippling or mottling, alternating light and dark spots of pigment loss and pigment clumping.

A classic example is the retinopathy of congenital rubella (Fig. 15a,b). Typically, there is fine to coarse pigment clumping or mottling. The changes may be generalized, or predominantly central or peripheral, unilateral or bilateral. The retinopathy may occur as the sole ocular stigmata of the disease, or in association with other ocular changes of congenital rubella such as cataract, glaucoma or microphthalmos. The retinal changes usually are stationary from birth and rarely progressive, although a late complication characterized by sudden macular hemorrhage and vision impairment may occur years after birth.

The pigmentary changes of syphilitic retinitis may also be of the 'salt and pepper' type.

Certain acquired viral exanthems of childhood, particularly rubeolla, also may produce fine pigmentary changes.

To be differentiated from the retinal pigmentary changes of infectious diseases are the retinal signs of certain metabolic disorders. The retinopathy of cystinosis, for example, is characterized by fine to coarse pigment clumping in an otherwise hypopigmented fundus (Fig. 15c). The pigment stippling commonly appears first in the periphery but in time may be seen throughout the fundus. As a rule it is not associated with vision loss. Important to the diagnosis, of course, is the detection of cystine crystals in the cornea and conjunctiva.

Also to be differentiated are certain retinal degenerations that may present with fine to coarse pigment mottling—such changes may be associated with progressive systemic or neurological disease (see p. 44) (Fig. 15d). Associated signs, progression and deterioration of function are, of course, crucial in the differential diagnosis of such conditions.

Not to be confused with 'salt and pepper' retinopathy is the pigment stippling often seen as a normal developmental variation in some blond and red-headed children.

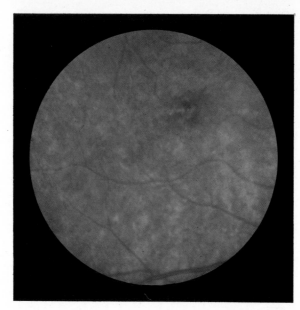

Figure 15a
'Salt and pepper' retinopathy
Note pattern of alternating light and dark spots, areas of depigmentation and pigment clumping. Child had congenital rubella syndrome.

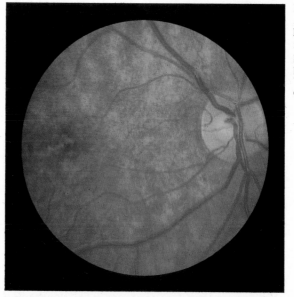

Figure 15b
Rubella retinopathy
In this child with congenital rubella there is coarse pigmentary mottling of posterior pole, and finer 'salt and pepper' stippling of other areas.

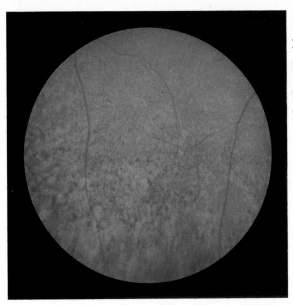

Figure 15c
Pigmentary retinopathy of cystinosis
The 'salt and pepper' pattern in this child is due to cystinosis. Retinopathy gave clue to diagnosis before corneal changes were documented by biomicroscopy.

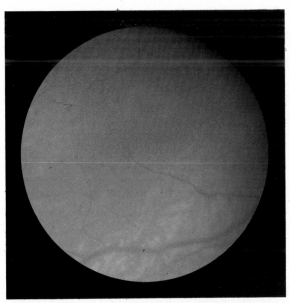

Figure 15d
Degeneration presenting with 'salt and pepper' changes
The coarse 'salt and pepper' type pigment changes in this infant with developmental delay, hypotonia and hepatomegaly, were the early manifestations of progressive neurological disease—Zellweger syndrome.

16 PIGMENTARY RETINAL DEGENERATION— RETINITIS PIGMENTOSA AND ITS VARIANTS

Pigmentary retinal degeneration is characterized by disorganization of the retinal pigmentary pattern, arteriolar attenuation, some degree of optic atrophy, and attendant impairment of visual function. Dispersion, migration and aggregation of retinal pigment produce a variety of ophthalmoscopically visible changes, ranging from fine granularity or coarse mottling to large focal aggregations of pigment with the configuration of bone spicules (Fig. 16a,b,c,d). The pigmentary changes usually appear first in the mid-periphery of the fundus, although in some cases the macula is affected first. Visual symptoms include impairment of dark adaptation, loss of peripheral field, often in the form of an expanding ring scotoma or concentric contraction of the visual field, and reduction of acuity. The ERG is reduced.

Pigmentary retinal degeneration may occur as an isolated ocular condition (classic 'retinitis pigmentosa'), as an inherited autosomal recessive, autosomal dominant, or sex-linked disorder; in association with other abnormalities as an expression of systemic, metabolic, or neurological disease; or as one feature of a multifaceted syndrome. It may be associated with polydactyly, obesity, hypogonadism and mental deficiency in the Laurence-Moon-Biedl syndrome; with abetalipoproteinemia and acanthocytosis as in the Bassen-Kornzweig syndrome; with progressive cerebellar ataxia and peripheral polyneuropathy in the Refsum syndrome; with hyperkinesia and mental retardation in Hallervorden-Spatz disease; or with progressive external ophthalmoplegia and heart block in the Kearns-Sayre syndrome. It can be a manifestation of generalized mucopolysaccharidosis, as in the syndromes of Hurler, Hunter, Scheie, and Sanfilippo, or as a manifestation of sphingolipidosis or lipofuscinosis, as in the syndromes of Batten-Mayou-Spielmeyer-Vogt or Jansky-Bielschowsky, to name just a few. Thus, in each case of pigmentary retinal degeneration consideration must be given to possible systemic, metabolic, neurological and genetic implications.

A type of pigmentary retinal degeneration or dystrophy of special importance in pediatrics is Leber's congenital amaurosis. In this condition the retinal changes are pleomorphic with varying degrees of pigment clumping and mottling. Severe vision impairment and an abnormal EEG are evident early.

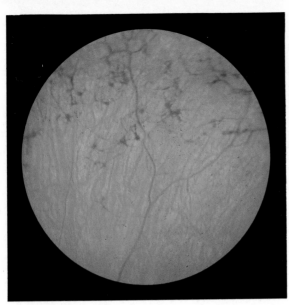

Figure 16a
Retinitis pigmentosa
These fundus changes are
typical of retinitis
pigmentosa. Note bone-
spicule pigment aggregates,
areas of pigment loss, and
arteriolar attenuation. This
otherwise healthy teenage
patient suffered progressive
vision loss beginning early
in childhood. Her siblings
were affected similarly.

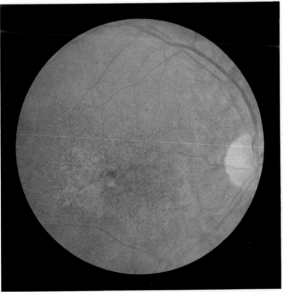

Figure 16b
Inverse retinitis pigmentosa
Subtle macular changes, disc
pallor and decreasing visual
acuity were first signs of
retinitis pigmentosa in this
otherwise normal eight-year-
old female. Classic
peripheral bone-spicule
pigment aggregates
developed in time.

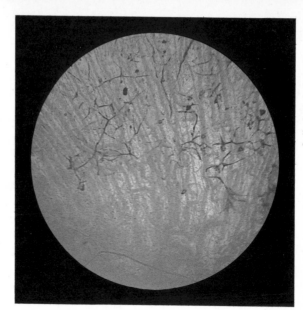

Figure 16c
Pigmentary retinal degeneration in ceroid lipofuscinosis
Retinitis pigmentosa-like changes developed late in childhood in this patient with ceroid lipofuscinosis. Child presented with seizures and progressive loss of abilities.

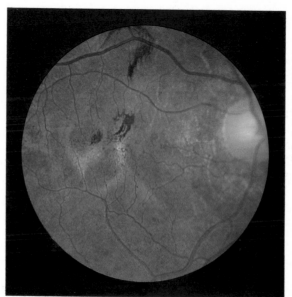

Figure 16d
Pigmentary retinal degeneration in a complex syndrome
These coarse retinal pigmentary changes and attendant vision loss occurred in an adolescent male with progressive external ophthalmoplegia, cerebellar ataxia and dementia (PEO-plus syndrome).

The term 'cherry-red spot' describes the clinically detectable macular changes produced when transparency of the retinal ganglion cells is lost, usually as the result of edema or lipid accumulation. On ophthalmoscopic examination, the multilayer ganglion-cell ring of the macula appears hazy or thickened, and of grayish, white or yellow color. In contrast to this pale or creamy halo, the vascular blush of the underlying choroid at the center of the macula, an area essentially devoid of ganglion cells, appears bright or dark red (Fig. 17a,b).

In pediatric practice, the macular cherry-red spot is most important as a sign of the neuronal lipidoses. It characteristically occurs in Tay-Sachs disease (GM_2 type 1) and in the Sandoff variant (GM_2 type 2); it also occurs in some cases of generalized gangliosidoses (GM_1 type 1). Cherry-red-like macular changes also have been described in other sphingolipidoses, particularly the neuronopathic forms of Niemann-Pick disease (sphingo-myelin lipidosis) and Gaucher disease (glucosyl ceramide lipidosis), in some cases of metachromatic leukodystrophy (sulfatide lipidosis) and in certain mucolipidoses, namely Farber disease and Spranger disease. However, the clinically visible macular changes in these conditions tend to be less well defined or more subtle than those of the classic cherry-red spot of Tay-Sachs disease.

It is to be remembered that in many diseases a cherry-red spot is only the focal, ophthalmoscopically visible macular sign of more widespread retinal or generalized neuronal degeneration.

To be differentiated from the cherry-red spot of neurodegenerative disease is the cherry-red spot that may occur as the result of retinal ischemia, as with occlusion of the central retinal artery, or in association with the retinal edema of ocular contusion (Fig. 17c).

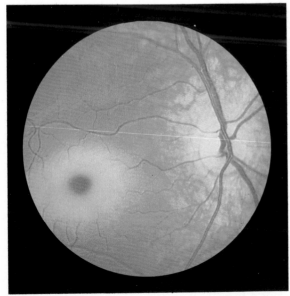

Figure 17a
Classical cherry-red spot
In this child with Tay-Sachs disease center of macula appears bright red in contrast to creamy pallor of macular ganglion-cell ring.

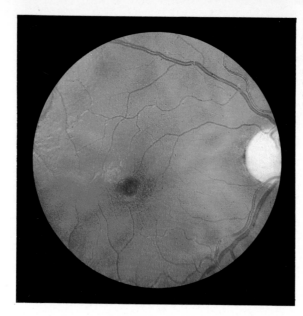

Figure 17b
Degenerated cherry-red spot
Over a period of years, the once brilliant cherry-red spot in this five-year-old child with Tay-Sachs disease degenerated, appearing 'burned-out'.

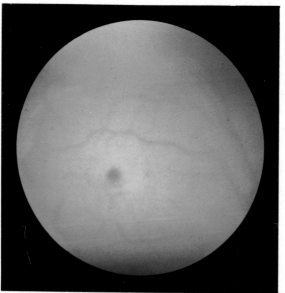

Figure 17c
Cherry-red spot of retinal ischemia
Unilateral cherry-red spot in this otherwise healthy 13-year-old girl was due to occlusion of central retinal artery. She suffered sudden loss of vision.

There are many types of macular degeneration with variation in the pathological features and clinical manifestations. Of major importance in pediatric practice are the hereditary degenerations. Some occur alone, as genetically determined primary macular or retinal disorders, without associated systemic or neurological involvement. Others occur in association with systemic or neurological signs, as manifestations of more widespread metabolic or neurodegenerative disease.

Two important types of heredomacular degeneration unassociated with central nervous system involvement are Stargardt's juvenile macular degeneration and Best vitelliform macular degeneration.

As originally described by Stargardt, juvenile macular degeneration is characterized by slowly progressive macular deterioration and attendant vision loss, manifesting by age eight to 20 years (Fig. 18a). Initially, there may be only mild changes of the pigment epithelium, a beaten-copper or beaten-silver appearance, and later a picture of more advanced atrophy of the pigment epithelium in the macular region. In some cases there are white or yellowish spots around the macula or throughout the posterior fundus, and there may be mild pigmentary changes in the periphery; in such cases the term fundus flavimaculatus is used (Fig. 18b). The ERG and peripheral fields usually are normal. The condition is autosomal recessive.

In Best vitelliform macular degeneration the characteristic lesion is a yellow or orange discoid subretinal macular lesion, resembling the intact yolk of a fried egg. This usually is diagnosed between ages five and 15 years, and as a rule the vision is normal in the early stage. The fundus signs, however, are variable. In some cases the macular abnormality is subtle, with minimal pigmentary changes or alteration of the foveal appearance. Often there is progressive macular degeneration characterized by atrophy, pigmentation, fibrous scarring, and attendant vision impairment. As a rule the ERG is normal; the EOG is abnormal in affected individuals and in carriers. This degeneration usually is autosomal dominant.

Macular degenerations associated with central nervous system degeneration commonly are referred to as the cerebromacular degenerations. This is a diverse group of disorders. Some are neuronal lipidoses (sphingolipidoses) in which the characteristic macular sign is a cherry-red spot; this important fundus sign is described separately (see p. 47). The prototype is Tay-Sachs disease. Others are the neuronal ceroid lipofuscinoses, sometimes classified for convenience as Batten disease or Batten-Vogt syndrome. Subclassification is based on age and clinical course, and includes (1) the infantile or Haltia-Santavuori type, (2) the late infantile, Jansky-Bielschowsky form, (3) the Spielmeyer-Vogt (or Mayou) type of juvenile or later-childhood onset, and (4) Kuf disease, the adult form.

In these Batten-type cerebromacular degenerations the earliest fundus sign is often dispersion, obtunding or loss of the foveal light reflex (Fig. 18c). Definition of the macular architecture may be lost, the macula may appear dull or take on a bull's-eye appearance. In time there may be signs of generalized retinal degeneration, including pigment disorder, arteriolar attenuation and optic atrophy (Fig. 18d).

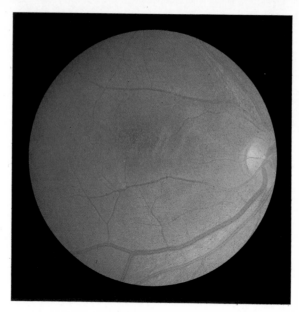

Figure 18a
Stargardt macular degeneration
Macular degeneration in this adolescent is characterized by dispersion of foveal light reflex and subtle pigment changes. Patient had no associated neurological signs.

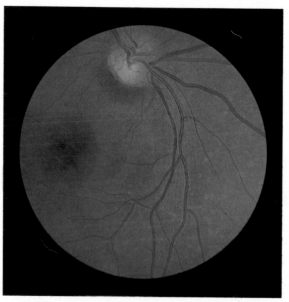

Figure 18b
Juvenile macular degeneration—flavimaculatus
This child with juvenile-onset macular degeneration also shows widespread retinal changes characteristic of fundus flavimaculatus.

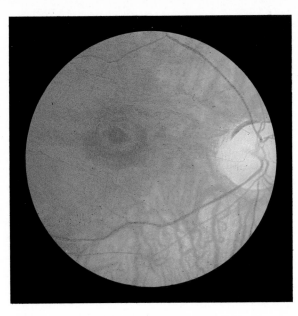

Figure 18c
Batten syndrome
In this child with progressive cerebroretinal degeneration, loss of foveal reflex and bull's-eye appearance of macula were early signs.

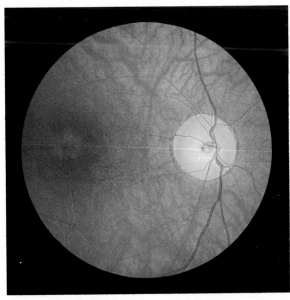

Figure 18d
Progressive macular degeneration
Note marked macular changes, arteriolar attenuation and optic atrophy in this child with late-onset cerebromacular degeneration (lipofuscinosis).

The term phakoma is derived from the Greek word for a mother spot or birthmark and is used to denote the herald lesions that occur in a number of the congenital hamartomatoses and neurocutaneous syndromes. Some of these herald lesions occur in the eye and their ophthalmoscopic appearance is often distinctive.

The characteristic ocular sign of tuberous sclerosis of Bourneville is an elevated, somewhat translucent or refractile, white to yellowish multi-nodular lesion of the retina or optic nervehead. The appearance of the classical lesion often is likened to that of an unripe mulberry (Fig. 19a). However, there is considerable variation in the fundus lesions of tuberous sclerosis; some are flat or only slightly elevated, dull yellow or white, and relatively smooth (Fig. 19b,c,d,e,f). The retinal lesions of tuberous sclerosis may be large or small, single or multiple, unilateral or bilateral. Histologically, they are benign astrocytic proliferations of the retina, often with cystic or calcific changes. A diligent search should be made for these tell-tale lesions in children with seizures, developmental delay and behavior disorders, with or without cutaneous signs such as adenoma sebaceum, mountain-ash leaf spots or shagreen patches.

In neurofibromatosis or von Recklinghausen disease, a retinal lesion similar to that of tuberous sclerosis may occur, but with less frequency. Another fundus sign in von Recklinghausen disease is abnormal pigmentation, likened to the café-au-lait spot of the skin. There may be disc changes, particularly optic atrophy or disc swelling of associated optic glioma, and ectopic medullation of the disc and retina occurs with somewhat increased frequency.

In addition to the fundus signs, nodular iris lesions, referred to as Lisch nodules, are important in the diagnosis of von Recklinghausen disease. There also may be neurofibromatous involvement of the lid (plexiform neuroma, ptosis) and orbit (proptosis, bony defects), or glaucoma.

In von Hippel-Lindau disease, or angiomatosis of the retina and cerebellum, the characteristic fundus lesion is a retinal hemangioblastoma. This is a globular vascular lesion that has the appearance of a toy balloon, with large paired vessels coursing to and from the lesion. In some cases the vascular changes are less conspicuous. Complications such as hemorrhage, exudation and retinal detachment may occur. The cerebellar lesion of von Hippel-Lindau disease may also produce papilledema and nystagmus, as well as ataxia.

In the Sturge-Weber syndrome of encephalofacial angiomatosis, the fundus sign is a choroidal hemangioma. This appears dark on ophthalmoscopic examination and fluoresces on angiography. Other significant fundus signs in this syndrome are tortuosity of the retinal vessels and anastamoses of the retinal veins. There may also be disc changes of intracranial hemorrhage and increased intracranial pressure. The more frequent and worrisome ocular complication of the Sturge-Weber disease, however, is glaucoma.

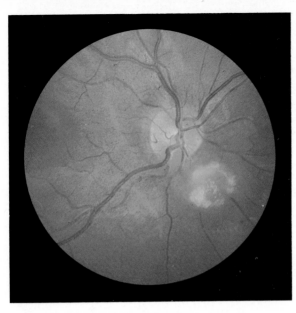

Figure 19a
Retinal phakoma
This refractile, elevated
multinodular lesion is
representative of classical
'mulberry' lesion of
tuberous sclerosis. Patient
also had typical adenoma
sebaceum.

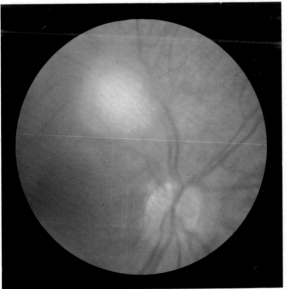

Figure 19b
Large hamartoma
Retinal phakoma in this
child is quite large and
smoothly elevated. Patient
presented with seizures and
retardation.

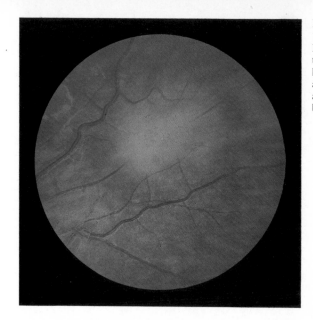

Figure 19c
Typical retinal phakoma
In many children with tuberous sclerosis, retinal lesions are relatively flat and somewhat translucent, as seen in this six-year-old boy.

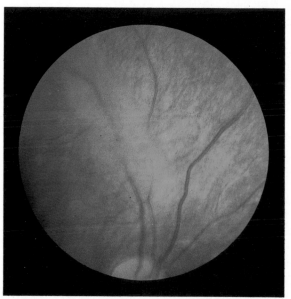

Figure 19d
Interesting variant
Translucent retinal phakoma in this one-year-old child with tuberous sclerosis extends several disc diameters along a major retinal vessel.

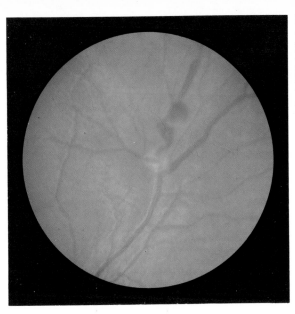

Figure 19e
Hamartoma with vessel abnormality
In this child with tuberous sclerosis a small retinal lesion is seen in association with sausage-like dilatation of retinal vessels.

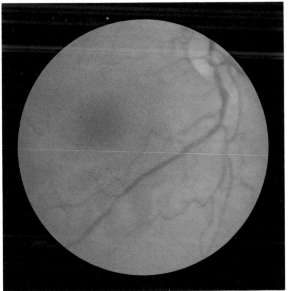

Figure 19f
Subtle lesion of tuberous sclerosis
Note small yellowish phakoma adjacent to inferotemporal vein in this seven-year-old child with seizures.

Retinoblastoma is a malignant tumor that arises from the retina. It occurs in hereditary, non-hereditary, and chromosomal deletion forms. It is primarily a tumor of childhood, usually appearing before five years of age, though rarely it may occur even in adults. One or both eyes can be affected.

Retinoblastoma may be single or multiple, large or small. On ophthalmoscopic examination the smaller tumors tend to appear as translucent thickening of the retina (Fig. 20). The larger tumors usually are more opaque and white. Feeder vessels and nodular chalky foci of calcification may be evident. Seeding into the vitreous is common. Some tumors grow diffusely into the vitreous as large masses (endophytic); others extend outward (exophytic) and may produce retinal detachment.

A frequent presenting sign is leukocoria, a white or 'cat's eye' reflex in the pupil. Another common sign is strabismus—deviation of the eye secondary to impairment of vision. Some children present with signs of ocular inflammation, intra-ocular hemorrhage, glaucoma or heterochromia iridis. Differential diagnosis includes simulating conditions such as persistent hyperplastic primary vitreous, retrolental fibroplasia, retinal dysplasia, and nematode endophthalmitis.

Retinoblastoma is a vision-threatening and potentially life-threatening tumor. There may be extension into the central nervous system or metastasis to other sites, particularly bone, liver, kidney and the adrenal glands. In addition some patients with retinoblastoma are at risk for other tumors, including osteogenic sarcoma, rhabdomyosarcoma and leukemia. Some may have concurrent brain tumor, particularly pinealoma. Thus detection, or even suspicion of retinoblastoma, is reason for prompt and thorough evaluation and treatment.

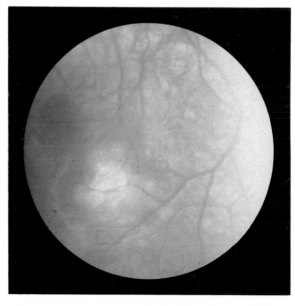

Figure 20
Retinoblastoma
Lesion, irregular in shape, is somewhat translucent, with opaque foci of calcification. Child, age nine months, also had an embryonal cell tumor of brain (suprasellar).

1 RETINOPATHY OF PREMATURITY (RETROLENTAL FIBROPLASIA)

This is a complex retinal vascular disorder that occurs primarily in infants whose retinas are incompletely vascularized at birth. At highest risk are infants born prematurely, particularly those of very low birthweight and those who have been seriously ill, requiring supplemental oxygen to sustain life and to prevent brain damage. It appears that in such infants the developing or immature retinal vasculature is vulnerable to potentially adverse effects of oxygen, and possibly other factors acting singly or in combination, that may result in the pathological changes and clinically significant alterations collectively referred to as retrolental fibroplasia (RLF) or the retinopathy of prematurity (ROP).

It should be recalled that normal retinal vasculogenesis proceeds from the disc to the periphery, usually reaching the ora serrata by 38 to 44 weeks. Mesenchyme, the vascular precursor tissue, grows across the retina and gives rise to a primitive capillary meshwork; this then undergoes active modeling to form more mature capillaries, arterioles and venules.

In ROP/RLF, two major abnormal processes or phases are recognized; (1) vaso-obliteration and (2) vasoproliferation. Studies indicate that upon exposure to oxygen* or during periods of relative hyperoxia, endothelial damage, closure and obliteration of developing retinal capillaries may occur. The mesenchyme that remains and the retinal arteries and veins that have already formed may then unite through surviving capillary channels to form a shunt. On ophthalmoscopic examination one may see the abrupt termination of the retinal vasculature, with a distinct line of demarcation between the vascularized retina and the nonvascularized peripheral zone (Fig. 21a). At this site the shunt may be seen as a discrete raised gray-white structure with fan-shaped arcades of vessels emptying into it. The vessels posterior to the shunt may be dilated and tortuous. The ischemic avascular retina, peripheral to the demarcation line, generally appears pale (gray, white), translucent or opaque and thickened. Proximal to the shunt there may be small vascular tufts or neovascular membranes projecting into the vitreous. There may also be retinal hemorrhages, exudates and some degree of retinal detachment.

The acute or active changes may continue for months after birth or terminate early. Fortunately, in many cases there is spontaneous regression of the retinopathy; the change is often marked by 'pinking-up' of the shunt and the beginning of the process of vascularization of the ischemic avascular zone.

Unfortunately, in others there is progressive overgrowth of vasoproliferative tissue into the vitreous, on the surface of the retina, over the ciliary body and around the back of the lens, with progressive cicatrization. Shrinkage of tissue can result in traction on the retina, dragging or folding of the retina (Fig. 21b), or detachment of the retina, and retinal pigmentary changes. All gradations of damage may occur, with varying degrees of vision impairment. In some cases the end result is total detachment of the retina, shallowing of the anterior chamber, hemorrhage,

---

*The precise levels of oxygen and period of exposure to oxygen sufficient to produce changes in susceptible infants have yet to be determined.

inflammation, secondary angle-closure glaucoma in a blind painful eye, or phthisis. There often is leukocoria, a white pupillary reflex arising from the retrolental tissue, the organized detachment, or from a secondary cataract.

There is often associated high myopia, a little-understood complication of cicatricial RLF, and a high incidence of strabismus and amblyopia.

To be differentiated from retinopathy of prematurity is familial exudative vitreoretinopathy, a disorder of the vitreous and retina that occurs as an autosomal dominant condition. It is characterized by the presence of organized membranes (often containing large blood vessels) in the vitreous, peripheral retinal exudation (subretinal and intraretinal), and in some cases localized retinal detachment and recurrent vitreous hemorrhages. The ocular changes are progressive and tend to run a downhill course.

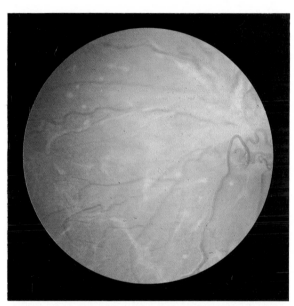

Figure 21a
Active ROP
Retinal edema and tortuosity of retinal vessels are evident.

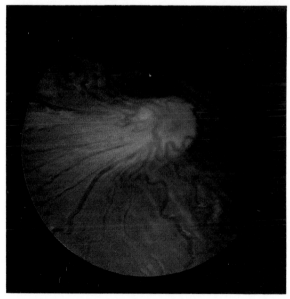

Figure 21b
'Dragged disc'
This picture is typical of cicatricial RLF. There is dragging of retina and retinal vessels to temporal side of disc.

The hallmark of hypertensive retinopathy is vasoconstriction. The vascular tone of the retinal artery increases by a process of autoregulation in response to the rise in blood pressure. On ophthalmoscopic examination one may see generalized arteriolar narrowing, focal arteriolar constriction ('spasm') with irregularity in the caliber of the vessels, and arterial tortuosity (Fig. 22a). Associated vessel damage and disruption of the blood-retinal barrier may occur, leading to leakage of plasma and formed blood elements in the retina. Clinically one may see retinal edema, hemorrhages and exudates (Fig. 22b). The hemorrhages typically are flame-shaped or splinter hemorrhages, as the extravasation of blood occurs primarily in the nerve-fiber layer. The exudates or edema residues appear yellow; those in the macula may form a star-shaped figure. In addition there may be superficial white spots called 'cotton-wool spots'; these are the result of focal ischemia and swelling of retinal-nerve fibers.

In time arteriolar sclerosis may occur. This is manifested by changes in the color of the arterioles, and changes in the arteriovenous crossings. As the vessel wall becomes 'harder' or 'thicker', the ophthalmoscopic reflection from the wall increases and the visibility of the blood column decreases; as sclerosis progresses the arteriole may take on a copper-wire appearance, or ultimately a silver-wire appearance. At arteriovenous crossings one may see obscuration of the venous blood column, deflection or change in the course of the vessels as they cross and, in some cases, signs of venous impedance (dilatation, tortuosity) distal to the crossing.

Another important manifestation of hypertension is hypertensive disc edema, characterized by swelling of the nervehead and blurring of the disc margins. This may occur with or without increased intracranial pressure of hypertensive encephalopathy. The pathogenesis is unclear, but alteration in the circulation to the optic nervehead and changes in tissue pressure and axoplasmic flow may occur in hypertension. Ischemia has been implicated as a factor.

In addition to the retinovascular and disc signs of hypertension there may be clinical signs of hypertensive choroidopathy, particularly in acute hypertension and in relatively young individuals. One may see changes in the retinal-pigment layer as a result of occlusive changes in the underlying choriocapillaries. Clinically, these appear as yellowish spots, or pigmented spots with depigmented halos, referred to as Elschnig spots.

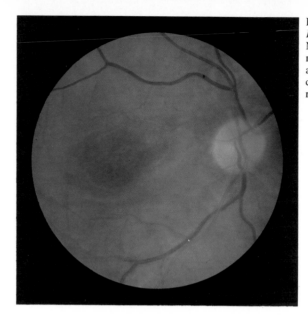

Figure 22a
Hypertensive retinopathy
Note generalized and focal
narrowing of retinal
arterioles, arteriovenous
crossing abnormality and
retinal edema.

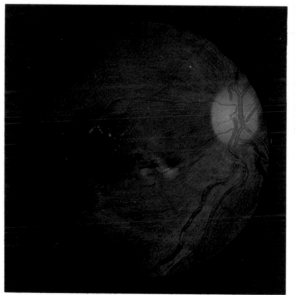

Figure 22b
Hypertensive retinopathy
In this child there are
marked hypertensive
changes including multiple
retinal hemorrhages,
exudates and prominent
alterations of the arterioles
and veins. (The fundus is
that of a black child; hence
the dark slate hue.)

60

The retinal manifestations of diabetes mellitus are classified as (1) simple or non-proliferative retinopathy, and (2) proliferative, the more severe type.

Non-proliferative or background retinopathy is characterized by venous dilatation, micro-aneurysms, retinal hemorrhages, exudates, cytoid bodies, and retinal edema (Fig. 23). The micro-aneurysms appear as tiny red dots; they often are the first detectable finding. The retinal hemorrhages may be of both the deep (intraretinal) dot and blot type, and the more superficial (nerve-fiber layer) splinter or flame-shaped type. The exudates tend to be deep and appear waxy. Cytoid bodies, descriptively referred to as cotton-wool spots, are superficial nerve-fiber infarcts. These background changes may wax and wane.

Proliferative retinopathy is characterized by neovascularization and proliferation of connective tissue on the retina and into the vitreous, often with vision-threatening complications such as retinal and vitreous hemorrhages, cicatrization, traction and retinal detachment. Rubeosis (abnormal vascularization of the iris) and secondary glaucoma may develop.

The incidence of diabetic retinopathy increases with duration of disease and with age. The incidence is low within the first five years of disease and increases thereafter. It is rare in prepubescent children, but its prevalence increases after puberty, rising noticeably after age 15 years. Examination of the fundus is important in the care of youngsters with diabetes.

In addition to retinal changes, patients with juvenile-onset diabetes may develop optic neuropathy, characterized by optic-disc edema with blurring of vision. They also may develop cataracts, sometimes of rapid onset.

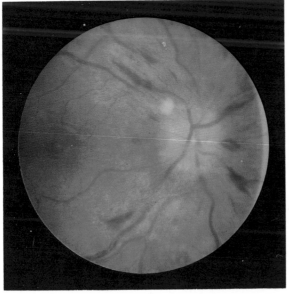

Figure 23
Diabetic retinopathy
Note multiple dot-like mirco-aneurysms, irregular dilatation of veins, splinter and flame-shaped hemorrhages, peripapillary cotton-wool spot and retinal edema. This girl's retinopathy developed at 16 years of age.

In various types of hyperlipoproteinemia there may be visible alteration in the color of the plasma. In some cases this change can be detected ophthalmoscopically, the blood column of the retinal vessels having a pale or creamy appearance (Fig. 24a); the term lipemia retinalis is used to describe this fundus sign.

The clinical picture can be dramatic, the creaminess being evident in vessels throughout the fundus; the fundus background may even appear pale, pink, or salmon colored. In some cases the change can be detected only in the smaller and more peripheral vessels where the blood column is thinner. Visibility of the lipemia may also vary with the transparency of the vessel walls, and the clarity of the ocular media.

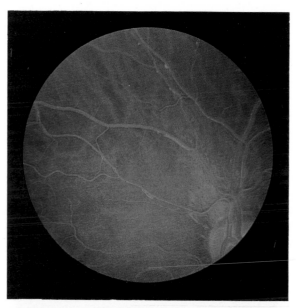

Figure 24a
Lipemia retinalis
Creamy alteration of blood column of retinal vessels is evident in this young girl with hyperlipidemia.

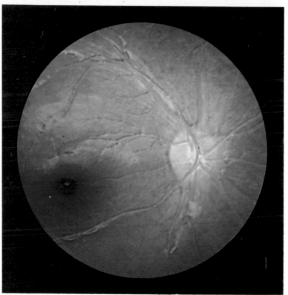

Figure 24b
Lipemia retinalis
Note milky pallor of fundus in addition to whitish lamination of blood-vessel column. This nine-year-old girl had hyperlipidemia and diabetes mellitus.

Lipemia retinalis is related to the level of triglycerides. It may occur in types I, III, IV or V hyperlipoproteinemia. In children with lipemia retinalis, type I (lipoprotein lipase deficiency) is the primary consideration; symptoms usually appear in the first decade. Lipemia retinalis may also be associated with diabetes mellitus (Fig. 24b).

Other ocular signs occurring with the various forms of hyperlipoproteinemia include xanthomas and corneal arcus.

25 ROTH SPOTS

Historically, this appellation has been used to denote the white-centered retinal hemorrhages seen in patients with subacute bacterial endocarditis, which were believed to be caused by septic emboli.

Similar in appearance, however, are the white-centered hemorrhages that occur in leukemia and a number of other systemic and ocular conditions, including ischemia, anoxia and anemia, diabetic and hypertensive retinopathy, and trauma, notably birth trauma and child abuse, to name just a few (Fig. 25). The white center in these hemorrhages is a fibrin thrombus.

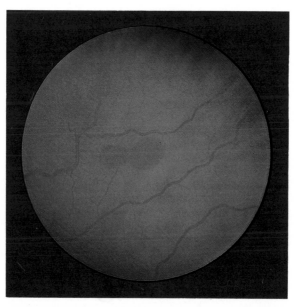

Figure 25
White-centered hemorrhage
Retinal hemorrhage with white center seen in this infant was due to trauma (child abuse).

The fundus signs of leukemia include dilatation, engorgement and tortuosity of the retinal veins, sheathing of the retinal vessels, retinal hemorrhages, exudates, cotton-wool spots, and nodular retinal infiltrates (Fig. 26). There may also be optic-nerve changes.

The dilatation of the veins is often irregular, producing a sausage-like appearance. The blood column may appear not only broad but pale, reflecting the increased white blood-cell content and the decreased red blood-cell content. In some cases there may be signs of venous obstruction.

Retinal hemorrhages are a frequent sign. They occur in all types of leukemia and are often present at the time of presentation or diagnosis. The retinal hemorrhages of leukemia are usually located in the posterior pole and in relationship to the retinal vessels. They may be of the superficial flame-shaped type, often with a white center, or of the deeper intraretinal round or blot type. Sometimes they are of the subhyaloid or so-called preretinal type, forming a fluid level and having the configuration of a boat keel. In some cases there is extravasation of blood into the vitreous, affecting vision and impairing visualization of the fundus.

Perivascular sheathing appears as a gray or white line along the vessel wall, resulting from diapedesis of the cells. There may also be localized aggregates of white cells, commonly referred to as leukemic nodules. These are to be differentiated from the exudates and cotton-wool patches (nerve-fiber infarcts) that may occur in leukemia.

With leukemic infiltration of the optic nerve one may see swelling of the nervehead, or a proliferative lesion, appearing as a fluffy or grayish mass protruding from the disc. With intracranial involvement, there may be papilledema of increased intracranial pressure.

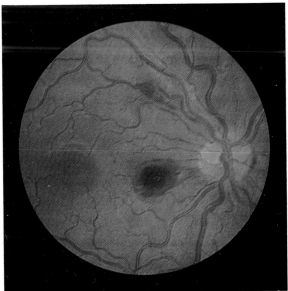

Figure 26
Leukemic retinopathy
In this child with acute lymphocytic leukemia, venous dilatation and tortuosity, and retinal hemorrhages are principal signs. Note small white spot in retinal hemorrhage, temporal to the disc.

The fundus signs, though frequent, are but a portion of the whole spectrum of leukemic ophthalmopathy. Other important manifestations are uveal involvement, notably iris infiltrates, hyphemia (bleeding into the anterior chamber), hypopyon (creamy layering of cells in the aqueous), lid, lacrymal and conjunctival infiltrates, and orbital masses. In addition one may see ocular complications of radiation therapy or evidence of ocular infection by opportunistic organisms.

RETINAL TELANGIECTASIS

Retinal telangiectasis, also referred to as Leber's miliary aneurysms, is a developmental vascular anomaly characterized by ophthalmoscopically visible, focal saccular dilatations of intraretinal capillaries, arterioles or venules (Fig. 27). The lesions usually are monocular, infrequently bilateral. There is propensity for temporal retinal location, though any area of the retina may be involved. The lesions occur in childhood and tend to be found primarily in adolescent males. The condition occasionally is familial. As a rule there are no regularly associated systemic lesions, though isolated instances of other abnormalities have been reported.

The extent and natural course of retinal telangiectasis is variable, but there is a tendency to intraretinal and subretinal exudation. This may lead to massive exudative detachment of the retina, often having a yellowish color, with attendant disturbance of vision, a condition referred to as Coats' disease. Such lesions may require treatment; ophthalmological evaluation and careful follow-up are indicated.

Not to be confused with congenital retinal telangiectasis is cavernous hemangioma of the retina, a hamartomatous condition characterized by a sessile hemangiomatous mass composed of clusters of saccular aneurysms of retinal vessels having the appearance of grapes projecting from the surface of the retina. It has been suggested that cavernous hemangioma of the retina and brain may occur together, and there may also be associated cutaneous lesions.

Also to be distinguished from retinal telangiectasis are aneurysmal changes of retina vessels that may occur with diabetes, venous stasis, macroglobulinemia, sickle-cell disease, or in association with angiomatosis retinae (von Hippel-Lindau disease, see p. 52), or racemose angioma, a very rare condition which may occur in association with arteriovenous malformation of the brain (Wyburn-Mason syndrome).

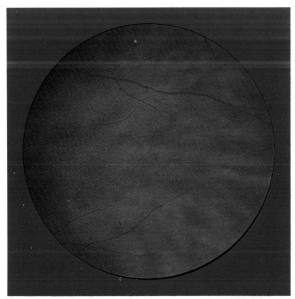

Figure 27
Retinal telangiectasis
Note multiple small grape-like aneurysmal lesions in the temporal fundus. Patient was an adolescent male referred for evaluation of learning disability. There were no associated systemic or neurological abnormalities.

Tortuosity of the retinal arterioles may occur as a benign congenital variant (Fig. 28). It may also occur as a familial disorder, and in some cases it may be associated with recurrent retinal hemorrhages and visual symptoms. The hemorrhages may be spontaneous or related to physical exertion. Usually there are no associated systemic abnormalities, though there may be a history of hemorrhages in other parts of the body.

To be differentiated from congenital retinal tortuosity is the tortuosity that may occur with hypertension, and this is an important sign in children with coarctation of the aorta. Also to be considered in the differential diagnosis of tortuosity are leukemia, polycythemia, macroglobulinemia, cryglobulinemia, sickle-cell disease, mucopolysaccharidosis (specifically Maroteaux-Lamy syndrome), and Fabry disease. Not to be confused with benign congenital retinal tortuosity are the retinal signs of Wyburn-Mason syndrome (racemose angioma of the retina and arteriovenous malformations of the brain) and of von Hippel-Lindau disease (angiomatosis retinae et cerebellae).

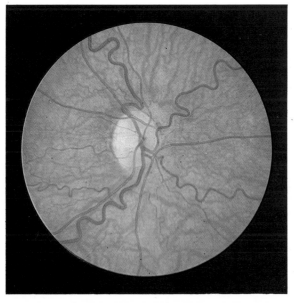

Figure 28
Retinal arteriolar tortuosity
Tortuosity of retinal artery in this child is a normal developmental variant.

In some individuals vascular loops may be seen projecting from the disc into the vitreous. The configuration may vary from that of a simple hairpin turn to a spiral, corkscrew, or figure-eight twist (Fig. 29). Some are surrounded by a sheath of whitish glial tissue. Some may be seen to pulsate. These are congenital anomalies. They are more often arterial than venous. They may be unilateral or bilateral.

In most cases prepapillary vascular loops present no problem, occurring just as interesting incidental findings in otherwise normal eyes. Occasionally, however, they may be associated with retinal vascular obstruction or hemorrhage.

Not to be confused with these simple congenital prepapillary vascular loops are more complex vascular anomalies, such as racemose angiomas that may be associated with arteriovenous malformations of the brain.

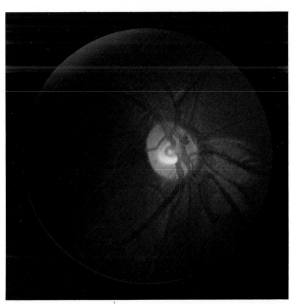

Figure 29
Prepapillary vascular loop
Note twisted loop of vessel projecting from disc. This is a developmental variant with no associated vascular or neurological signs in this child.

Hypopigmentation of the fundus is a not-uncommon finding and presents a number of diagnostic possibilities. Though marked hypopigmentation of the fundus may be seen as a normal developmental variant in many blond individuals, especially in infants and young children, pigment deficiency can be an important manifestation of metabolic disease. Of primary importance in the differential diagnosis of pathological fundus hypopigmentation are the various forms of albinism.

In oculocutaneous albinism there is generalized hypopigmentation of the skin, hair and eyes. The iris typically is pale blue or gray and translucent. The fundus appears pale and red-streaked owing to absence of background pigmentation and increased visibility of the underlying sclera and choroidal vasculature (Fig. 30a). In addition there is hypoplasia of the macula—it appears flat with poor definition of the ganglion-cell ring and foveal light-reflex, and the disc also may appear pale, grayish and somewhat hypoplastic. Vision is subnormal, there is nystagmus, and the patient is sensitive to light. High refractive errors and strabismus are frequent associated findings.

Tyrosinase negative and tyrosinase positive forms of oculocutaneous albinism can be differentiated; these are recessive. An Amish or yellow variant, having a different enzyme defect, also occurs; ocular signs are similar and persist throughout life, though some skin color develops.

Incomplete forms of albinism also occur and an important example is ocular albinism. In this condition hypopigmentation is limited to the eye. The condition is most commonly x-linked and pigment disorder of the fundus may be seen in carrier females.

Important syndromes associated with various forms of albinism are the Hermansky-Pudlak syndrome, the Chediak-Higashi syndrome, and the Cross syndrome. The Hermansky-Pudlak syndrome is an autosomal recessive condition characterized by oculocutaneous albinism and a hemorrhagic diathesis. The Chediak-Higashi syndrome is characterized by incomplete oculocutaneous albinisim, neutropenia, and susceptibility to pyogenic infections. The Cross syndrome is characterized by hypopigmentation, gingival fibromatosis, spasticity, athetoid movements, and microphthalmos.

To be considered in the differential diagnosis of partial albinism is Waardenburg syndrome; this autosomal dominant condition is characterized primarily by poliosis, heterochromia, telecanthus, and hearing impairment.

It is of interest that children with cystinosis or Menke's trichopoliodystrophy may also have a markedly hypopigmented or albinotic fundus (Fig. 30b).

To be differentiated from the developmental disorders affecting pigmentation are the degenerative diseases characterized by loss of pigment, such as retinitis pigmentosa and choroideremia.

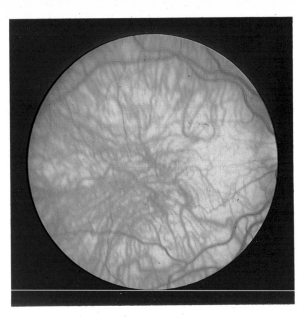

Figure 30a
Albinism
This child with oculocutaneous albinism shows the classical findings of generalized hypopigmentation of the fundus with increased visibility of the choroidal vascular pattern.

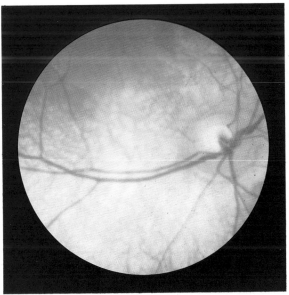

Figure 30b
Albinotic fundus
Marked hypopigmentation of fundus seen here is in a child with Menke's trichopoliodystrophy, a complex metabolic neurodegenerative disease.

This disorder is characterized by the presence of multiple yellow-white spots in the retina in association with congenital stationary night-blindness. The fundus spots are small (about the size of a second-order arteriole) and extend from the posterior pole to the periphery (Fig. 31a,b).

To be distinguished from fundus albipunctatus is retinitis punctata albescens, a degenerative disorder characterized by progressive visual-field loss, retinal pigmentary changes and arteriolar attenuation.

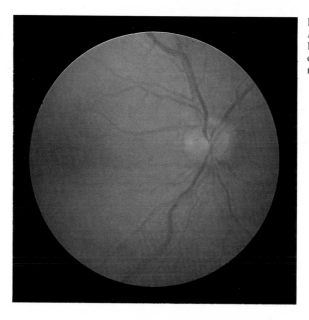

Figure 31a
Fundus albipunctatus
Note punctate yellow spots of retina. Retinal vessels are normal.

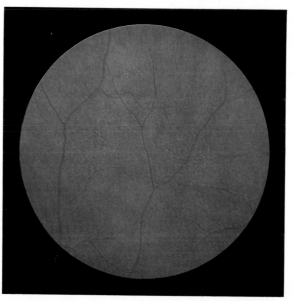

Figure 31b
Fundus albipunctatus
Typical yellow punctate lesions are seen throughout periphery.

SELECTED READING

Papilledema

Barr C. C., Glaser, J. S., Blankenship, G. (1980) 'Acute disc swelling in juvenile diabetes. Clinical profile and natural history of 12 cases.' *Archives of Ophthalmology*, **98**, 2185-2192.

Billson F. A., Hudson, R. L. (1975) 'Surgical treatment of chronic papillodema in children.' *British Journal of Ophthalmology*, **59**, 92-95.

Buchheit, W. A., Burton, C., Haag, B., Shaw, D. (1969) 'Papilledema and idiopathic intracranial hypertension. Report of a familial occurrence.' *New England Journal of Medicine*, **280**, 938-942.

Hayreh, S. S. (1977) 'Optic disc edema in raised intracranial pressure. V. Pathogenesis.' *Archives of Ophthalmology*, **95**, 1553-1565.

Hayreh, S. S. (1977) 'Optic disc edema in raised intracranial pressure. VI. Associated visual disturbances and their pathogenesis.' *Archives of Ophthalmology*, **95**, 1566-1579.

Pavan, P. R., Aiello, L. M., Wafai, M. Z., Briones, J. C., Sebestyen, J. G., Bradbury, M. J. (1980) 'Optic disc edema in juvenile-onset diabetes.' *Archives of Ophthalmology*, **96**, 2193-2195.

Rosenberg, M. A., Savino, P. J., Glaser, J. S. (1979) 'A clinical analysis of pseudopapilledema. I. Population, laterality, acuity, refractive error, ophthalmoscopic characteristics, and coincident disease.' *Archives of Ophthalmology*, **97**, 65-70.

Savino, P. J., Glaser, J. S., Rosenberg, M. A. (1979) 'A clinical analysis of pseudopapilledema. II. Visual field defects.' *Archives of Ophthalmology*, **97**, 71-75.

Optic neuritis

Frey, T. (1973) 'Optic neuritis in children. Infectious mononucleosis as an etiology.' *Documenta Ophthalmologica*, **34**, 183-188.

Godel, V., Nemet, P., Lazar, M. (1980) 'Chloramphenicol optic neuropathy.' *Archives of Ophthalmology*, **98**, 1417-1421.

Harley, R. D., Huang, N. N., Macri, C. H., Green, W. R. (1970) 'Optic neuritis and optic atrophy following chloramphenicol in cystic fibrosis patients.' *Transactions of the American Academy of Ophthalmology and Otolaryngology*, **74**, 1011-1031.

Kazarian, E. L., Gager, W. E. (1978) 'Optic neuritis complicating measles, mumps, and rubella vaccination.' *American Journal of Ophthalmology*, **86**, 544-547.

Kennedy, C., Carroll, F. D. (1960) 'Optic neuritis in children.' *Archives of Ophthalmology*, **63**, 747-755.

Kennedy, C., Carter, S. (1961) 'Relation of optic neuritis to multiple sclerosis in children.' *Pediatrics*, **28**, 377-387.

Meadows, S. R. (1969) 'Retrobulbar and optic neuritis in childhood and adolescence.' *Transactions of the Ophthalmological Society of the United Kingdom*, **89**, 603-638.

Selbst, R. G., Selhorst, J. B., Harrison, J. W., Myer, E. C. (1983) 'Parainfectious optic neuritis. Report and review following varicella.' *Archives of Neurology*, **40**, 347-350.

Smith, J. L., Hoyt, W. F., Susac, J. D. (1973) 'Ocular fundus in acute Leber optic neuropathy.' *Archives of Ophthalmology*, **90**, 349-354.

Strong, L. E., Henderson, J. W., Gangitano, J. L. (1974) 'Bilateral retrobulbar neuritis secondary to mumps.' *American Journal of Ophthalmology*, **78**, 331-332.

Optic atrophy

Blodi, F. C. (1957) 'Developmental anomalies of the skull affecting the eye.' *Archives of Ophthalmology*, **57**, 593-610.

Davis, W. H., Nevins, R. C., Elliott, J. H. (1972) 'Optic atrophy after ocular contusion.' *American Journal of Ophthalmology*, **73**, 278-280.

Fishman, M. L., Bean, S. C., Cogan, D. G. (1976) 'Optic atrophy following prophylactic chemotherapy and cranial radiation for acute lymphocytic leukemia.' *American Journal of Ophthalmology*, **82**, 571-576.

Hoyt, C. S. (1980) 'Autosomal dominant optic atrophy. A spectrum of disability.' *Ophthalmology*, **87**, 245-251.

Kline, L. B., Glaser, J. S. (1979) 'Dominant optic atrophy. The clinical profile.' *Archives of Ophthalmology*, **97**, 1680-1686.

Kollarits, C. R., Pinheiro, M. L., Swann, E. R., Marcus, D. F., Corrie, W. S. (1979) 'The autosomal dominant syndrome of progressive optic atrophy and congenital deafness.' *American Journal of Ophthalmology*, **87**, 789-792.

Nikoskelainen, E., Sogg, R. I., Rosenthal, A. R., Friberg, T. R., Dorfman, L. J. (1977) 'The early phase in Leber hereditary optic atrophy.' *Archives of Ophthalmology*, **95**, 969-978.

Schwartz, J. F., Chutorian, A. M., Evans, R. A., Carter, S. (1964) 'Optic atrophy in childhood.' *Pediatrics*, **34**, 670-679.

Wybar, K. C. (1972) 'Acquired optic atrophy in early childhood.' *In* Cant, J. S. (Ed.) *The Optic Nerve*. London: Henry Kimpton; St. Louis: C. V. Mosby. pp. 12-18.

Optic-cup enlargement

Armaly, M. F. (1967) 'Genetic determination of cup/disc ratio of the optic nerve.' *Archives of Ophthalmology*, **78**, 35-43.

Armaly, M. F. (1969) 'The optic cup in the normal eye. I. Cup width, depth, vessel displacement, ocular tension and outflow facility.' *American Journal of Ophthalmology*, **68**, 401-407.

Khodadoust, A. A. Ziai, M., Biggs, S. L. (1968) 'Optic disc in normal newborns.' *American Journal of Ophthalmology*, **66**, 502-504.

Richardson, K. T., Shaffer, R. N. (1966) 'Optic-nerve cupping in congenital glaucoma.' *American Journal of Ophthalmology*, **62**, 507-509.

Robin, A. L., Quigley, H. A., Pollack, I. P., Maumenee, A. E., Maumenee, I. H. (1979) 'An analysis of visual acuity, visual fields, and disk cupping in childhood glaucoma.' *American Journal of Ophthalmology*, **88**, 847-858.

Optic-nerve pits

Brown, G. C., Shields, J. A., Goldberg, R. E. (1980) 'Congenital pits of the optic nerve head. II. Clinical studies in humans.' *Ophthalmology*, **87**, 51-65.

Pfaffenbach, D. D., Walsh, F. B. (1972) 'Central pit of the optic disk.' *American Journal of Ophthalmology*, **73**, 102-106.

Optic-nerve hypoplasia

Brook, C. G. D., Sanders, M. D., Hoare, R. D. (1972) 'Septo-optic dysplasia.' *British Medical Journal*, **3**, 811-813.

Krause-Brucker, W., Gardner, D. W. (1980) 'Optic nerve hypoplasia associated with absent septum pellucidum and hypopituitarism.' *American Journal of Ophthalmology*, **89**, 113-120.

Layman, P. R., Anderson, D. R., Flynn, J. T. (1974) 'Frequent occurrence of hypoplastic optic disks in patients with aniridia.' *American Journal of Ophthalmology*, **77**, 513-516.

Mosier, M. A., Lieberman, M. F., Green, W. R., Knox, D. L. (1978) 'Hypoplasia of the optic nerve.' *Archives of Ophthalmology*, **96**, 1437-1442.

Petersen, R. A., Walton, D. S. (1977) 'Optic nerve hypoplasia with good visual acuity and visual field defects. A study of children of diabetic mothers.' *Archives of Ophthalmology*, **95**, 254-258.

Skarf, B., Hoyt, C. S. (1984) 'Optic nerve hypoplasia in children. Association with anomalies of the endocrine and CNS.' *Archives of Ophthalmology*, **102**, 62-67.

Walton, D. S., Robb, R. M. (1970) 'Optic nerve hypoplasia. A report of 20 cases.' *Archives of Ophthalmology*, **84**, 572-578.

Weiter, J. J., McLean, I. W., Zimmerman, L. E. (1977) 'Aplasia of the optic nerve and disk.' *American Journal of Ophthalmology*, **83**, 569-576.

Tilted disc

Graham, M. V., Wakefield, G. J. (1973) 'Bitemporal visual field defects associated with anomalies of the optic discs.' *British Journal of Ophthalmology*, **57**, 307-314.

Hittner, H. M., Borda, R. P., Justice, J. (1981) 'X-linked recessive congenital stationary night blindness, myopia, and tilted discs.' *Journal of Pediatric Ophthalmoplegia and Strabismus*, **18**, 15-20.

Young, S. E., Walsh, F. B., Knox, D. L. (1976) 'The tilted disk syndrome.' *American Journal of Ophthalmology*, **82**, 16-23.

Optic-disc drusen

Frisén, L., Schöldström, G., Svendsen, P. (1978) 'Drusen in the optic nerve head. Verification by computerized tomography.' *Archives of Ophthalmology*, **96**, 1611-1614.

Harris, M. J., Fine, S. L., Owens, S. L. (1981) 'Hemorrhagic complications of optic nerve drusen.' *American Journal of Ophthalmology*, **92**, 70-76.

Sanders, T. E., Gay, A. J., Newman, M. (1971) 'Hemorrhagic complications of drusen of the optic disk.' *American Journal of Ophthalmology*, **71**, (Suppl.) 204-217.

Spencer, W. H. (1978) 'Drusen of the optic disk and aberrant axoplasmic transport.' *American Journal of Ophthalmology*, **85**, 1-12.

Tso, M. O. M. (1981) 'Pathology and pathogenesis of drusen of the optic nervehead.' *Ophthalmology*, **88**, 1066-1080.

Persistent Bergmeister papilla

Lloyd, R. I. (1940) 'Variations in the development and regression of Bergmeister's papilla and the hyaloid artery.' *Transactions of the American Ophthalmological Society*, **38**, 326-332.

Roth, A. M., Foos, R. Y. (1972) 'Surface structure of the optic nerve head. Epipapillary membranes.' *American Journal of Ophthalmology*, **74**, 977-985.

Persistent hyperplastic primary vitreous (PHPV)
Brown, G. C., Gonder, J., Levin, A. (1984) 'Persistence of the primary vitreous in association with the morning glory disc anomaly.' *Journal of Pediatric Ophthalmology and Strabismus,* **21,** 5-7.
Federman, J., Shields, J. A., Altman, B., Koller, H. (1982) 'The surgical and non-surgical management of persistent hyperplastic primary vitreous.' *Ophthalmology,* **89,** 20-24.
Goldberg, M. F., Mafee, M. (1983) 'Computed tomography for diagnosis of persistent hyperplastic primary vitreous (PHPV).' *Ophthalmology,* **90,** 442-451.
Haddad, R., Font, R. L., Reeser, F. (1978) 'Persistent hyperplastic primary vitreous: a clinico-pathologic study of 62 cases and review of the literature.' *Survey of Ophthalmology,* **23,** 123-124.
Pruett, R. C., Schepens, C. L. (1970) 'Posterior hyperplastic primary vitreous.' *American Journal of Ophthalmology,* **69,** 535-543.
Reese, A. B. (1955) 'Persistent hyperplastic primary vitreous.' *American Journal of Ophthalmology,* **40,** 317-331.

Myelinated nerve fibers
Holland, P. M., Anderson, B. (1976) 'Myelinated nerve fibers and severe myopia.' *American Journal of Ophthalmology,* **81,** 597-599.
Straatsma, B. R., Heckenlively, J. R., Foos, R. Y., Shahinian, J. K. (1979) 'Myelinated retinal nerve fibers associated with ipsilateral myopia, ambylopia and strabismus.' *American Journal of Ophthalmology,* **88,** 506-510.
Straatsma, B. R., Foos, R. Y., Heckenlively, J. R., Taylor, G. N. (1981) 'Myelinated retinal nerve fibers.' *American Journal of Ophthalmology,* **91,** 25-38.

Peripapillary crescents
Shields, M. B. (1980) 'Gray crescent in the optic nerve head.' *American Journal of Ophthalmology,* **89,** 238-244.

Colobomata
Francois J. (1968) 'Colobomatous malformations of the ocular globe.' *International Ophthalmological Clinics,* **8,** 797-817.
Goldhammer, Y., Smith, J. L. (1975) 'Optic nerve anomalies in basal encephalocele.' *Archives of Ophthalmology,* **93,** 115-118.
Hittner, H. M., Desmond, M. M., Montgomery, J. R. (1976) 'Optic nerve manifestations of human congenital cytomegalovirus infection.' *American Journal of Ophthalmology,* **81,** 661-665.
James, P. M. L., Karseras, A. G., Wybar, K. C. (1974) 'Systemic associations of uveal coloboma.' *British Journal of Ophthalmology,* 58, 917-921.
Kindler, P. (1970) 'Morning glory syndrome. Unusual congenital optic disc anomaly.' *American Journal of Ophthalmology,* **69,** 376-384.
Koenig, S. B., Naidich, T. P., Lissner, G. (1982) 'The morning glory syndrome associated with sphenoidal encephalocoele.' *Ophthalmology,* **89,** 1368-1373.
Pagon, R. A., Graham, J. M., Zonana, J., Young, S. L. (1981) 'Coloboma congenital heart disease, and choanal atresia with multiple anomalies. CHARGE association.' *Journal of Pediatrics,* **99,** 223-227.
Savell, J., Cook, J. R. (1976) 'Optic nerve coloboma of autosomal-dominant heredity.' *Archives of Ophthalmology,* **94,** 395-400.

Chorioretinitis
Asbell, P. A., Vermund, S. H., Hopelot, A. J. (1982) 'Presumed toxoplasmic retinochoroiditis in four siblings.' *American Journal of Ophthalmology,* **94,** 656-663.
Charles, N. C., Bennett, T. W., Margolis, J. I. (1977) 'Ocular pathology of the congenital varicella syndrome.' *Archives of Ophthalmology,* **95,** 2034-2037.
Chumbley, L. C., Kearns, T. P. (1972) 'Retinopathy of sarcoidosis.' *American Journal of Ophthalmology,* **73,** 123-131.
Cibis, G. W., Flynn, J. T., Davis, E. B. (1978) 'Herpes simplex retinitis.' *Archives of Ophthalmology,* **96,** 299-302.
Cogan, D. G. (1977) 'Immunosuppression and eye disease.' *American Journal of Ophthalmology,* **83,** 777-788.
Cogan, D. G., Kuwabara, T., Young, G. F., Knox, D. L. (1964) 'Herpes simplex retinopathy in an infant.' *Archives of Ophthalmology,* **72,** 641-645.
Cox, F., Meyer, D., Hughes, W. T. (1975) 'Cytomegalovirus in tears from patients with normal eyes and with acute cytomegalovirus chorioretinitis.' *American Journal of Ophthalmology,* **80,** 817-824.
Desmonts, G., Couvreue, J. (1974) 'Toxoplasmosis in pregnancy and its transmission to the fetus.' *Bulletin of the New York Academy of Medicine,* **50,** 146-159.

Duguid, I. M. (1961) 'Features of ocular infestation by *Toxocara.' British Journal of Ophthalmology*, **45,** 789-796.

Fine, S. L., Owens, S. L., Haller, J. A., Knox, D. L., Patz, A. (1981) 'Choroidal neovascularization as a late complication of ocular toxoplasmosis.' *American Journal of Ophthalmology*, **91,** 318-322.

Gould, H., Kaufman, H. E. (1961) 'Sarcoid of the fundus.' *Archives of Ophthalmology*, **65,** 453-456.

Hagler, W. S., Walters, P. V., Naumias, A. J. (1969) 'Ocular involvement in neonatal Herpes simplex virus infection.' *Archives of Ophthalmology*, **82,** 169-176.

Hogan, M. J., Kimura, S. J., Spencer, W. H. (1965) 'Visceral larva migrans and peripheral retinitis.' *Journal of the American Medical Association*, **194,** 1345-1347.

Knox, D. L., (1983) 'Disorders of the uveal tract.' *In* Harley, R. D. (Ed.) *Pediatric Ophthalmology, 2nd Edn.* Philadelphia: W. B. Saunders.

Lonn, L. I. (1972) 'Neonatal cytomegalic inclusion disease chorioretinitis.' *Archives of Ophthalmology*, **88,** 434-438.

Martyn, L. J., Lischner, H. W., Pileggi, A. J., Harley, R. D. (1972) 'Chorioretinal lesions in familial chronic granulomatous disease of childhood.' *American Journal of Ophthalmology*, **72,** 403-418.

Molk, R. (1983) 'Ocular toxocaiasis: a review of the literature.' *Annals of Ophthalmology*, **15,** 216-231.

Pollard, Z. F. (1979) 'Ocular toxocara in siblings of two families. Diagnosis confirmed by Elisa test.' *Archives of Ophthalmology*, **97,** 2319-2320.

Smith, M. E., Zimmerman, L. E., Harley, R. D. (1966) 'Ocular involvement in congenital cytomegalic inclusion disease.' *Archives of Ophthalmology*, **76,** 696-699.

Smith, R. E., Ganley, J. P. (1972) 'Presumed ocular histoplasmosis. I. Histoplasmin skin test sensitivity in cases identified during a community survey.' *Archives of Ophthalmology*, **87,** 245-250.

Zimmerman, L. (1961) 'Ocular pathology of toxoplasmosis.' *Survey of Ophthalmology*, **6,** 832-839.

'Salt and pepper' retinopathy

Bateman, J. B., Riedner, E. D., Levin, L. S., Maumenee, I. N. (1980) 'Heterogeneity of retinal degeneration and hearing impairment syndromes.' *American Journal of Ophthalmology*, **90,** 755-767.

Boniuk, M., Zimmerman, L. E. (1967) 'Ocular pathology in the rubella syndrome.' *Archives of Ophthalmology*, **77,** 455-473.

Deutman, A. F., Grizzard, W. S. (1978) 'Rubella retinopathy and subretinal neovascularization.' *American Journal of Ophthalmology*, **85,** 82-87.

Hertzberg, R. (1968) 'Twenty-five-year follow-up of ocular defects in congenital rubella.' *American Journal of Ophthalmology*, **66,** 269-271.

Krill, A. E. (1967) 'The retinal disease of rubella.' *American Journal of Ophthalmology*, **77,** 445-449.

Scheie, H. G., Morse, P. H. (1972) 'Rubeola retinopathy.' *Archives of Ophthalmology*, **88,** 341-344.

Wong, V. G. (1976) 'Ocular manifestations in cystinosis.' *Birth Defects. Original Article Series*, **XII,** 181-186.

Pigmentary retinal degeneration

Bateman, J. B., Riedner, E. D., Levin, L. S., Maumenee, I. H. (1980) 'Heterogeneity of retinal degeneration and hearing impairment syndromes.' *American Journal of Ophthalmology*, **90,** 755-767.

Berson, E. L., Rosner, B., Simonoff, E. (1980) 'Risk factors for genetic typing and detection in retinitis pigmentosa.' *American Journal of Ophthalmology*, **89,** 763-775.

Edwards, W. C., Grizzard, W. S. (1981) 'Tapeto-retinal degeneration associated with renal disease.' *Journal of Pediatric Ophthalmology and Strabismus*, **18,** 55-57.

Eller, W. E., Brown, G. C. (1984) 'Retinal disorders of childhood.' *American Journal of Ophthalmology*, **98,** 1099-1101.

Fishman, G. A., Maggiano, J. M., Fishman, M. (1983) 'Foveal lesions seen in retinitis pigmentosa.' *Archives of Ophthalmology*, **95,** 1993-1996.

Gartner, S., Henkind, P. (1982) 'Pathology of retinitis pigmentosa.' *Ophthalmology*, **89,** 1425-1432.

Harcourt, B., Hopkins, D. (1972) 'Tapetoretinal degeneration in childhood presenting as a disturbance of behaviour.' *British Medical Journal*, **1,** 202-205.

Hittner, H. M., Zeler, R. S. (1975) 'Ceroid-lipofuscinosis (Batten disease). Fluorescein angiography, electrophysiology, histopathology, ultrastructure, and a review of amaurotic familial idiocy.' *Archives of Ophthalmology*, **98,** 178-183.

Koerner, F., Schlote, W. (1972) 'Chronic progressive external ophthalmoplegia. Association with retinal pigmentary changes and evidence in favor of ocular myopathy.' *Archives of Ophthalmology*, **88**, 155-166.

Marmor, M. F., Aguirre, G., Arden, G., Berson, E., Birch, D. G., Boughman, J. A., Carr, R., Chatrian, G. E., Del Monte, M., Dowling, J., Enoch, J., Fishman, G. A., Fulton, A. B., Garcia, C. A., Gouras, P., Heckenlively, J., Hu, D., Lewis, R. A., Niemeyer, G., Parker, J. A., Perlman, I., Ripps, H., Sandberg, M. A., Siegel, I., Weleber, R. G., Wolf, M. L., Wu, L., Young, R. S. L. (1983) 'Retinitis pigmentosa. A symposium on terminology and methods of examination.' *Ophthalmology*, **90**, 126-131.

McKusick, V. A., Neufeld, E. F., Kelly, T. E. (1978) 'The mucopolysaccharide storage diseases.' *In* Stanbury, J. B., Wyngaarden, J. B., Fredrickson, D. S. (Eds.) *The Metabolic Basis of Inherited Disease, 4th Edn.* New York: McGraw-Hill. pp. 1282-1307.

Newell, F. W., Johnson, R. O., Huttenlocher, P. R. (1979) 'Pigmentary degeneration of the retina in the Hallervorden-Spatz syndrome.' *American Journal of Ophthalmology*, **88**, 467-471.

Noble, K. G., Carr, R. E. (1978) 'Leber's congenital amaurosis. A retrospective study of 33 cases and a histopathological study of one case.' *Archives of Ophthalmology*, **96**, 818-821.

Pearlman, J. T., Flood, T. P., Seiff, S. R. (1977) 'Retinitis pigmentosa without pigment.' *American Journal of Ophthalmology*, **81**, 417-419.

Peterson, W. S., Albert, D. M. (1974) 'Fundus changes in the hereditary nephropathie.' *Transactions of the American Academy of Ophthalmology and Otolaryngology*, **78**, 762-771.

Seiff, S. R., Heckenlively, J. R., Pearlman, J. T. (1982) 'Assessing the risk of retinitis pigmentosa with age-of-onset data.' *American Journal of Ophthalmology*, **94**, 38-43.

Yee, R. D., Herbert, P. N., Bergsma, D. R., Biemer, J. J. (1976) 'Atypical retinitis pigmentosa in familial hypobetalipoproteinemia.' *American Journal of Ophthalmology*, **82**, 64-71.

Cherry-red spot

Brownstein, S., Carpenter, S., Polomeno, R. C., Little, J. N. (1980) 'Sandnoff's disease (Gm_2 gangliosidosis type 2) histopathology and ultrastructure of the eye.' *Archives of Ophthalmology*, **98**, 1089-1097.

Cogan, D. G. (1966) 'Ocular correlates of inborn metabolic defects.' *Canadian Medical Association Journal*, **95**, 1055-1065.

Cogan, D. G., Chu, F. C., Gittinger, J., Tyschen, L. (1980) 'Fundal abnormalities of Gauchner's disease.' *Archives of Opthalmology*, **98**, 2202-2203.

Cotlier, E. (1971) 'Tay-Sachs' retina: deficiency of acetyl nexosaminidase A.' *Archives of Ophthalmology*, **86**, 352-356.

Emery, J. M., Green, W. R., Wyllie, R. G., Nowell, R. R. (1971) 'Gm_1-gangliosidosis, ocular and pathological manifestations.' *Archives of Ophthalmology*, **85**, 179-187.

Emery, J. M., Green, W. R., Huff, D. S., Sloan, H. R. (1972) 'Niemann-Pick disease (type C): histopathology and ultrastructure.' *American Journal of Ophthalmology*, **74**, 1144-1154.

Goldberg, M. F., Cotlier, E., Fichenscher, L. G., Kenyon, K., Enat, R., Borowsky, S. A. (1971) 'Macular cherry-red spot, corneal clouding, and β-galactosidase deficiency; clinical, biochemical, and electron microscopic study of a new autosomal recessive storage disease. *Archives of International Medicine*, **128**, 387-398.

Libert, J., Van Hoof, F., Toussaint, D., Roozitalab, H., Kenyon, K. P., Green, W. R. (1979) 'Ocular findings in metachromatic leukodystrophy. An electron microscopic and enzyme study in different clinical and genetic variants.' *Archives of Ophthalmology*, **97**, 1495-1504.

Rapin, I. (1976) 'Ocular correlates of inborn metabolic defects.' *Canadian Medical Association Journal*, **95**, 1055-1065.

Walton, D. S., Robb, R. M., Crocker, A. E. (1978) 'Ocular manifestations of group A Niemann-Pick disease.' *American Journal of Ophthalmology*, **85**, 174-180.

Macular degeneration

Barricks, M. E. (1977) 'Vitelliform lesions developing in normal fundi.' *American Journal of Ophthalmology*, **83**, 324-327.

Beckerman, B. L., Rapin, I. (1975) 'Ceroid lipofuscinosis.' *American Journal of Ophthalmology*, **80**, 73-77.

Carr, R. E., Noble, K. G. (1980) 'Juvenile macular degeneration.' *Ophthalmology*, **87**, 83-85.

Cibis, G. W., Morey, M., Harris, D. J. (1980) 'Dominantly inherited macular dystrophy with flecks (Stargardt).' *Archives of Ophthalmology*, **98**, 1785-1789.

Eagle, R. C., Lucier, A. C., Bernardino, V. B., Yanoff, M. (1980) 'Retinal pigment epithelial abnormalities in fundus flavimaculatus.' *Ophthalmology*, **87**, 1189-1200.

Gravina, R. F., Nakanishi, A. S., Faden, A. (1978) 'Subacute sclerosing panencephalitis.' *American Journal of Ophthalmology*, **86**, 106-109.

Hadden, O. B., Gass, J. D. M. (1976) 'Fundus flavimaculatus and Stargardt's disease.' *American Journal of Ophthalmology*, **82,** 527-539.

Krill, A. E. (1973) 'Juvenile macular degenerations. Part I.' *Ophthalmology Digest*, April 1973, 37-42.

Krill, A. E. (1973) 'Juvenile macular degnerations. Part II.' *Ophthalmology Digest*, May 1973, 33-40.

Krill, A. E., Morse, P. A., Potts, A. M., Klein, B. A. (1966) 'Hereditary vitelliform macular degeneration.' *American Journal of Ophthalmology*, **61,** 1405-1415.

Noble, K. G., Carr, R. (1979) 'Stargardt's disease and fundus flavimaculatus.' *Archives of Ophthalmology*, **97,** 1281-1285.

Schochet, S. S., Font, R. L., Morris, H. H. (1980) 'Jansky-Bielschowsky form of neuronal ceroid-lipofuscinosis.' *Archives of Ophthalmology*, **98,** 1083-1088.

Phakomata

Alexander, G. L., Norman, R. M. (1960) *The Sturge-Weber Syndrome*. Bristol: John Wright. pp. 1-87.

Cotlier, E. (1977) 'Cafe-au-lait spots of the fundus in neurofibromatosis.' *Archives of Ophthalmology*, **95,** 1990-1992.

Grover, W. D., Harley, R. D. (1969) 'Early recognition of tuberous sclerosis by funduscopic examination.' *Journal of Pediatrics*, **75,** 991-995.

Hardwig, P., Robertson, D. M. (1984) 'von Hippel-Lindau disease: a familial, often lethal multi-system phakomatosis.' *Ophthalmology*, **91,** 263-270.

Horowitz, P. (1971) 'von Hippel-Lindau disease.' *In* Tasman, W. (Ed.) *Retinal Diseases in Children*. New York: Harper & Row. pp. 78-91.

Kirby, T. J. (1951) 'Ocular phakomatoses.' *American Journal of Medical Sciences*, **222,** 227-239.

Lagos, J. C., Gomez, M. R. (1967) 'Tuberous sclerosis: reappraisal of a clinical entity.' *Mayo Clinical Proceedings*, **42,** 26-49.

Lewis, R. A., Riccardi, V. M. (1981) 'von Recklinghausen neurofibromatosis. Incidence of iris hamartomata.' *Ophthalmology*, **88,** 348-354.

Lloyd, L. A. (1973) 'Gliomas of the optic nerve and chiasma in childhood.' *Transactions of the American Ophthalmological Society*, **71,** 488-535.

Miller, S. J. H. (1963) 'Ophthalmic aspects of the Sturge-Weber syndrome.' *Proceedings of the Royal Society of Medicine*, **56,** 419-423.

Nyboer, J. H., Robertson, D. M., Gomez, M. R. (1976) 'Retinal lesions in tuberous sclerosis.' *Archives of Ophthalmology*, **94,** 1277-1280.

Riley, F. C., Campbell, R. J. (1979) 'Double phakomatosis.' *Archives of Ophthalmology*, **97,** 518-520.

Salazar, F. G., Lamiell, J. M. (1980) 'Early identification of retinal angiomas in a large kindred with von Hippel-Lindau disease.' *American Journal of Ophthalmology*, **89,** 540-545.

Retinoblastoma

Char, D. H. (1980) 'Current concepts in retinoblastoma.' *Annals of Ophthalmology*, **12,** 792-804.

Dryja, T. P., Cavenee, W., White, R., Rapaport, J. M., Petersen, R., Albert, D. M., Bruns, G. A. P. (1984) 'Homozygosity of chromosome 13 in retinoblastoma.' *New England Journal of Medicine*, **310,** 550-553.

Gallie, B. L., Phillips, R. A. (1984) 'Retinoblastoma: a model of oncogenesis.' *Ophthalmology*, **91,** 666-672.

Howard, G. M., Ellsworth, R. M. (1965) 'Differential diagnosis of retinoblastoma. A statistical survey of 500 children. I. Relative frequency of the lesions which simulate retinoblastoma.' *American Journal of Ophthalmology*, **60,** 610-618.

Lopez, J. F.-V., Alvarez, J. C. (1983) 'Atypical echographic forms of retinoblastoma.' *Journal of Pediatric Ophthalmology and Strabismus*, **20,** 230-234.

Margo, C. E., Zimmerman, L. E. (1983) 'Retinoblastoma: the accuracy of clinical diagnosis in children treated by enucleation.' *Journal of Pediatric Ophthalmology and Strabismus*, **20,** 227-229.

Murphree, A. L., Benedict, W. F. (1984) 'Retinoblastoma: clues to human oncogenesis.' *Science*, **223,** 1028-1033.

Shields, J. A., Augsburger, J. J. (1981) 'Current approaches to the diagnosis and management of retinoblastoma.' *Survey of Ophthalmology*, **25,** 347-372.

Zimmerman, L. E., Burns, R. P., Wankum, G., Tully, R., Esterly, J. A. (1982) 'Trilateral retinoblastoma: ectopic intracranial retinoblastoma associated with bilateral retinoblastoma.' *Journal of Pediatric Ophthalmology and Strabismus*, **19,** 320-325.

Retinopathy of prematurity (retrolental fibroplasia)

Ashton, N. (1979) 'The pathogenesis of retrolental fibroplasia.' *Ophthalmology*, **86**, 1695-1699.

Brockhurst, R. J., Albert, D. M., Zakov, Z. N. (1981) 'Pathologic findings in familial exudative vitreoretinopathy.' *Archives of Ophthalmology*, **99**, 2143-2146.

Criswick, V. G., Schepens, C. L. (1969) 'Familial exudative vitreoretinopathy.' *American Journal of Ophthalmology*, **68**, 578-594.

Finer, N. N., Schindler, R. F., Peters, K. I., Grant, G. D. (1983) 'Vitamin E and retrolental fibroplasia. Improved visual outcome with early vitamin E.' *Ophthalmology*, **90**, 428-435.

Flynn, J. T., Cassady, J., Essner, D., Zeskind, J., Merritt, J., Flynn, R., Williams, M. J. (1979) 'Fluorescein angiography in retrolental fibroplasia: experience from 1969-1977.' *Ophthalmology*, **86**, 1700-1723.

Gow, J., Oliver, G. L. (1971) 'Familial exudative vitreoretinopathy. An expanded view.' *Archives of Ophthalmology*, **86**, 150-154.

Gunn, T. R., Easdown, J., Outerbridge, E. W., Aranda, J. V. (1980) 'Risk factors in retrolental fibroplasia.' *Pediatrics*, **65**, 1096-1100.

Palmer, E. A. (1981) 'Optimal timing of examination for acute retrolental fibroplasia.' *Ophthalmology*, **88**, 662-668.

Patz, A. (1983) 'Current therapy of retrolental fibroplasia, retinopathy of prematurity.' *Ophthalmology*, **90**, 425-427.

Schulman, J., Jampol, L. M., Schwartz, N. (1980) 'Peripheral proliferative retinopathy without oxygen therapy in a full-term infant.' *American Journal of Ophthalmology*, **90**, 509-514.

Slusher, M. M., Hutton, W. E. (1979) 'Familial exudative vitreoretinopathy.' *American Journal of Ophthalmology*, **87**, 152-156.

Tasman, W. (1979) 'Late complications of retrolental fibroplasia.' *Ophthalmology*, **86**, 1724-1740.

Hypertensive retinopathy

Tso, M. O. M., Jampol, L. M. (1982) 'Pathophysiology of hypertensive retinopathy.' *Ophthalmology*, **89**, 1132-1145.

Walsh, J. B. (1982) 'Hypertensive retinopathy. Description, classification and prognosis.' *Ophthalmology*, **89**, 1127-1131.

Diabetic retinopathy

Barr, C. C., Glaser, J. S., Blankenship, G. (1980) 'Acute disc swelling in juvenile diabetes. Clinical profile and natural history of 12 cases.' *Archives of Ophthalmology*, **98**, 2185-2192.

Frank, R. N., Hoffman, W. H., Podgor, M. J., Joondeph, H. C., Lewis, R. A., Margherio, R. R., Nachazel, D. P., Weiss, H., Christopherson, K. W., Cronin, M. A. (1980) 'Retinopathy in juvenile-onset diabetes of short duration.' *Ophthalmology*, **87**, 1-9.

Jackson, R. L., Ide, C. H., Guthrie, R. A., James, R. D. (1982) 'Retinopathy in adolescents and young adults with onset of insulin-dependent diabetes in childhood.' *Ophthalmology*, **89**, 7-13.

Noble, K. G., Carr, R. E. (1983) 'Diabetic retinopathy. I. Nonproliferative retinopathy.' *Ophthalmology*, **90**, 1261-1263.

Lipemia retinalis

Kurz, G. H., Shakib, M., Sohmer, K. K., Friedman, A. H. (1976) 'The retina in type 5 hyperlipoproteinemia.' *American Journal of Ophthalmology*, **82**, 32-43.

Vinger, P. F., Sachs, B. A. (1970) 'Ocular manifestations of hyperlipoproteinemia.' *American Journal of Ophthalmology*, **70**, 563-573.

Roth spots

Duane, T. D., Osher, R. H., Green, W. R. (1980) 'White centered hemorrhages: their significance.' *Ophthalmology*, **87**, 66-69.

Phelps, C. D. (1971) 'The association of pale-centered retinal hemorrhages with intracranial bleeding in infancy.' *American Journal of Ophthalmology*, **72**, 348-350.

Leukemic retinopathy

Allen, R. A., Straatsma, B. R. (1961) 'Ocular involvement in leukemia and allied disorders.' *Archives of Ophthalmology*, **66**, 490-508.

Chalfin, A. I., Nash, B. M., Goldstein, J. H. (1973) 'Optic nervehead involvement in lymphocytic leukemia.' *Journal of Pediatric Ophthalmology*, **10**, 39-43.

Holt, J. M., Gordon-Smith, E. C. (1969) 'Retinal abnormalities in diseases of the blood.' *British Journal of Ophthalmology*, **53**, 145-160.

Ridgeway, E. W., Jaffe, N., Walton, D. S. (1976) 'Leukemic ophthalmopathy in children.' *Cancer*, **38**, 1744-1749.

Rosenthal, A. R. (1983) 'Ocular manifestations of leukemia.' *Ophthalmology*, **90**, 899-905.

Retinal telangiectasis

Archer, D. B. (1971) 'Leber's miliary aneurysms.' *Ophthalmology Digest,* July 1971, 8-13.

Farkas, T. G., Potts, A. M., Boone, C. (1973) Some pathologic and biochemical aspects of Coats' disease.' *American Journal of Ophthalmology,* **75,** 289-301.

Gass, J. D. M. (1971) 'Cavernous hemangioma of the retina: a neuro-cutaneous syndrome.' *American Journal of Ophthalmology,* **71,** 799-814.

Gass, J. D., Oyakawaw, R. T. (1982) 'Idiopathic juxtafoveolar retinal telangiectasis.' *Archives of Ophthalmology,* **100,** 769-780.

Goldberg, R. E., Pheasant, T. R., Shields, J. A. (1979) 'Cavernous hemangioma of the retina. A four-generation pedigree with neurocutaneous manifestations and an example of bilateral retinal involvement.' *Archives of Ophthalmology,* **97,** 2321-2324.

Reese, A. B. (1956) 'Telangiectasis of the retina and Coat's disease.' *American Journal of Ophthalmology,* **42,** 1-8.

Retinal arteriolar tortuosity

Goldberg, M. F., Pollack, I. P., Green, W. R. (1972) 'Familial retinal arteriolar tortuosity with retinal hemorrhage.' *American Journal of Ophthalmology,* **73,** 183-191.

Prepapillary vascular loops

Brown, G. C., Magargal, L., Augsburger, J. J., Shields, J. A. (1979) 'Preretinal arterial loops and retinal arterial occlusion.' *American Journal of Ophthalmology,* **87,** 646-651.

Degenhart, W., Brown, G. C., Augsburger, J. J., Magargal, L. (1981) 'Prepapillary vascular loops. A clinical and fluorescein angiographic study.' *Ophthalmology,* **88,** 1126-1131.

Albinotic fundus

Bergsma, D. R., Kaiser-Kupfer, M. (1974) 'A new form of albinism.' *American Journal of Ophthalmology,* **77,** 837-844.

Creel, D., O'Donnell, F. E., Witkop, C. J. (1978) 'Visual system anomalies in human ocular albinos.' *Science,* **102,** 931-933.

diGeorge, A. M., Ounsted, R. W., Harley, R. D. (1960) 'Waardenburg syndrome.' *Journal of Pediatrics,* **57,** 649-669.

Falls, H. F. (1953) 'Albinism.' *Transactions of the American Academy of Ophthalmology and Otolaryngology,* **57,** 324-331.

Hittner, H. M., King, R. A., Riccardi, V. M., Ledbetter, D. H., Borda, R. P., Ferrell, R. E., Kretzer, F. L. (1982) 'Oculocutaneous albinoidism as a manifestation of reduced neural crest derivatives in the Prader-Willi syndrome.' *American Journal of Ophthalmology,* **94,** 328-337.

O'Donnell, F. E., Hambrick, G. W., Green, W. R., Iliff, W. J., Stone, D. L. (1976) 'X-linked ocular albinism. An oculocutaneous macromelanosomal disorder.' *Archives of Ophthalmology,* **94,** 1883-1892.

O'Donnell, F. E., King, R. A., Green, W. R., Witkop, C. J. (1978) 'Autosomal recessively inherited ocular albinism. A new form of ocular albinism affecting females as severely as males.' *Archives of Ophthalmology,* **96,** 1621-1626.

Simon, J. W., Adams, R. J., Calhoun, J. H., Shapiro, S. S., Ingerman, C. M. (1982) 'Ophthalmic manifestations of the Hermansky-Pudlak syndrome (oculocutaneous albinism and hemorrhagic diathesis).' *American Journal of Ophthalmology,* **93,** 71-77.

Fundus albipunctatus

Carr, R. E., Margolis, S., Siegel, I. M. (1984) 'Fluorescein angiography and vitamin A and oxalate levels in fundus albipunctatus.' *American Journal of Ophthalmology,* **82,** 549-558.

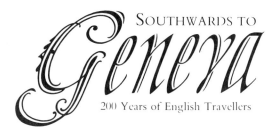

SOUTHWARDS TO

Geneva

200 Years of English Travellers

Leo and Anne,
With love and all possible
good wishes from
Mavis

Southwards to
Geneva

200 Years of English Travellers

—— MAVIS COULSON ——

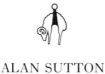

ALAN SUTTON
1988

ALAN SUTTON PUBLISHING
BRUNSWICK ROAD · GLOUCESTER

First published 1988

British Library Cataloguing in Publication Data

Coulson, Mavis
Southwards to Geneva.
1. Switzerland. Geneva. Intellectual
life, history
I. Title
949.4'5

ISBN 0-86299-509-4

Jacket: view of Geneva from
Saint-Antoine in 1815, attributed to
Ferrière (*Photograph: Nicolas Bouvier*)

Typesetting and origination by
Alan Sutton Publishing Limited
Printed in Great Britain

*To John – a
constantly-supportive husband
who has shared the Genevan
experience.*

CONTENTS

ACKNOWLEDGEMENTS

This book would not have seen the light of day without the help of many Genevan friends and well-wishers. First, I should like to express my warmest thanks to the Fonds Rapin for their generous grant. Then, I want to make particular mention of Jean-Flavien Lalive and Francine Long, whose efforts as 'midwives' to my English Travellers have gone far beyond the call of friendship and will always be remembered. Gerda Bouvier, also, has devoted many hours of research to further this project; and I have been fortunate enough to have had the advice and help of Nicolas Bouvier. To all these friends, and to others who have helped speed the book on its way, my very appreciative thanks!

I have had help and co-operation from many museums. Above all, I should like to thank Mme. Jacqueline Congnard, of the Musée d'art et d'histoire in Geneva, for her generous help and support. I am also most grateful to M. Michel Piller, of the Bibliothèque Publique et Universitaire and to M. Muti, of the Musée Tavel. My thanks are also due to the Courtauld Institute and the Whitworth Art Gallery, Manchester. The chapter-head engravings are from *Nouveaux Voyages en Zigzag* by Rodolphe Töpffer.

Finally, I want to express gratitude to Dorothy Middleton for her initial warm interest, to Elaine Robson-Scott for her meticulous reading of the proofs, and to Eliane Wilson, for constant encouragement and advice.

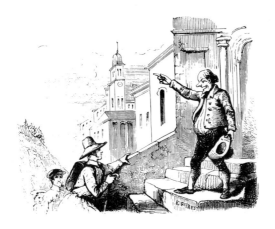

PREFACE

For today's air-traveller to Geneva, arrival can be dramatically beautiful. The aircraft seems to float in a sea of cloud, lit dazzlingly by sunlight. Here and there, mountain peaks rise through the cloud-waves like snow-capped volcanoes, and you cannot mistake the enormous mass of Mount Blanc. All is dreamlike and, as in a dream, there is no supporting structure. Now the plane begins to dive. Gradually the cocoon of swirling cloud falls away and, suddenly, there is Lac Leman – blue with mountain intensity – its shores eyelashed with small villages and quaysides. As the pilot flies lower, towards the south-west corner of the lake, you see the slopes below the Jura mountains chequered with small vineyards. Here and there a little turretted *manoir* straddles a hill and as the plane nears Geneva the lakeside becomes peppered with substantial villas. Snow-capped, the Alps march along the high horizon to the south – culminating in the massif of Mount Blanc sprawling far above the world. The plane is now flying close to the water and, before it comes in to land, you have a brief glimpse of Geneva itself: small yachts jostling in tiny ports; the feathered plume of the famous *jet d'eau* soaring high above the fringing houses; the deep-green Rhône sliding out of the lake; a gleaming shopping-centre on either side of the water, linked by bridges; and the Old Town, clustered round the spire of St Pierre, rising behind.

What, then, is Geneva today? One thing is certain: this twentieth-century town, with its charming waterfront and medieval quarter, is very much more than a pretty face. The town and canton are vibrant with activity of all kinds: private bankers,

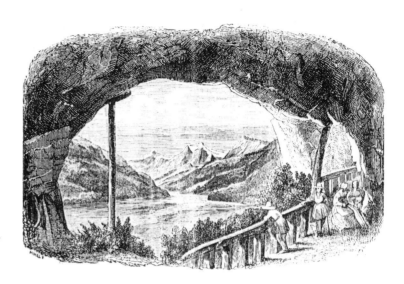

La Grotte de Balme by
Rudolfe Töpffer (from
Voyages en Zizgag)

international lawyers, jewellers, watch-makers, salesmen
marketing every device for pleasure-making, medical researchers,
doctors, university scholars and, above all, a mass of international
organisations (within and without the United Nations' umbrella)
teeming with international ants. Faced with such a mammoth
foreign invasion, it is small wonder that the Genevese of today
suffer from xenophobia. How else can they preserve their
identity?

This they have certainly achieved and the Genevese families of
today bear the names of their forebears who welcomed our
English travellers in the past. Pictets, Turettinis, Lullins, Bou-
viers, Sarasins, de Saussures, Hentsches, de Candolles, Cramers:
these names and others, prominent in today's Geneva, are the
same as those which recur again and again in the past – and in the
following pages.

Drawing by Rodolphe
Töpffer (from
*Nouveaux Voyages en
Zigzag*)

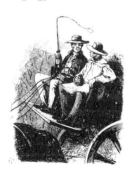

Before looking more closely at Geneva as it appeared to those
visiting Englishmen of the seventeenth and eighteenth centuries,
it seems of value to glance briefly at the general background.
Switzerland and its Alps have exercised a fascination for the
Englishman ever since the seventeenth century. Indeed, Weber[1]
observed that in the second half of the eighteenth century 'Of
twenty guests in a Swiss Inn it was usual to find that fourteen
were English'.

In 1818 von Haller writes, somewhat damningly:

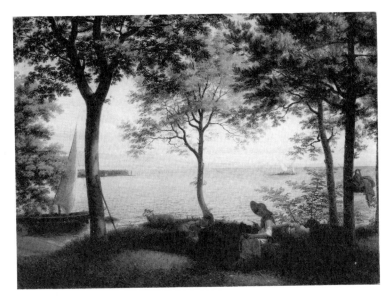

Beside the Lake at
Sécheron by Charles-
Joseph Auriol, 1822.
(*Collection Musée d'art
et d'histoire, Geneva*)

These foreign guests [English Tourists] do not realise that
. . . prices must naturally be higher in the mountains . . . In
addition, they are niggardly, hard, arrogant, and exuberant;
they bargain and give no tips even for extra and particular
services; they overwork horses and guides, show no
consideration for the innkeeper when his house is full, dirty
the linen unduly and show the most unfounded distrust
everywhere.[2]

John Murray's first *Handbook on Switzerland*, published in
1838, also gives, regrettably, a less than flattering picture of both
the Swiss peasant and the English traveller who made use of his
amenities.

With regard to the natural beauties of Switzerland, there can
be but one sentiment of admiration. On the subject of the
moral condition of the Swiss, and of their character as a
nation, there is much greater variety of opinion . . . The
poverty of the land, its slight capabilities for improvements,
its deficiency of resources in proportion to the extent of its
population, have given rise to that venality of character
which has passed into a proverb . . .

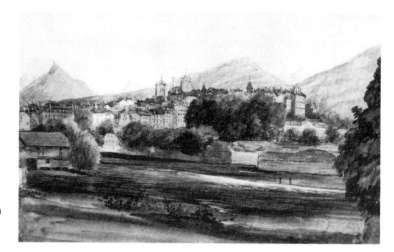

View from the Bastion
of Saint Jean, Geneva,
artist unknown, *c.* 1840
(*Collection Musée d'art
et d'histoire, Geneva*)

At a later stage, Murray quotes from Latrobe's *Alpenstock*:

It cannot be denied that the character of the majority of the
Swiss peasantry, whose habitations are unfortunately in the
neighbourhood of the main routes of travellers . . . is most
contemptible . . . The writer . . . must candidly add . . .
that the absurd conduct and unreasonable folly of travellers
have strengthened the spring of . . . dishonest propensity in
a very great degree . . .

And having been rude to the Swiss, Latrobe proceeds to
castigate his own countrymen:

Drawing by Rodolphe
Töpffer (from
*Nouveaux Voyages en
Zigzag*)

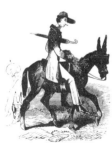

I have seen a party of English arrive at a mountain cabaret at
nightfall, when the host and his family would, in the usual
course of things, have been thinking of their beds; they order
dinner, and insist upon having flesh, fish, or fowl, foreign
wines and liqueurs, just as though they were at the Star and
Garter at Richmond; abuse the master and the domestics,
dine at eight or nine, and sit over their cheer till past
midnight. Mine host can put up with a good deal of extra
trouble, with no small quantity of abuse, and will stay up all
night with considerable temper, because he knows he can
make them pay for it in hard money . . .

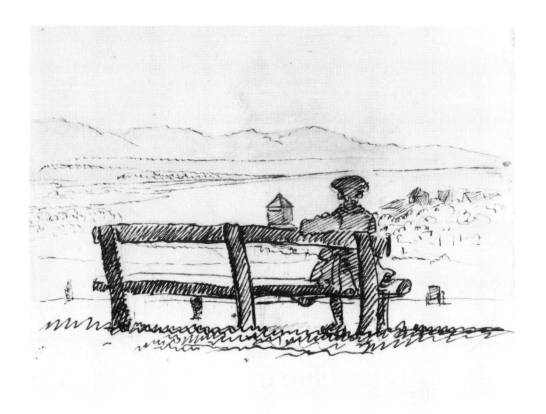

Man seen from behind looking at Lake Geneva, by Huber the Elder, 1765 (*Collection Musée d'art et d'histoire, Geneva*)

Be that as it may, the fact is that more and more Englishmen and women have found their way to Switzerland during the past three hundred years – partly in connection with the Grand Tour, partly for a variety of other reasons. Against this background, Geneva has always provided its own Mecca, for throughout the last three centuries the English have gravitated to this small Calvinist republic in their thousands – indeed probably in their tens of thousands.

But what originally drew them in such numbers? What was it they hoped to find? Did they come by chance or design? What was their relationship with their hosts? It is hoped that the following pages provide answers to some of these questions, though with such a plethora of available material, there can be no attempt to be comprehensive. From time to time, I have singled out some English character, be he or she artist or writer, for closer scrutiny. I have also included, exceptionally, a more detailed study of one Genevese personality, in order to highlight aspects of the intellectual life which served as a strong link between England and Geneva. Where religion and politics are concerned, I have not gone into very great detail. Had I done so, there would have been little time for anything else, and I have intentionally stretched my canvas between the mid-seventeenth century and the mid-Victorian period in order to avoid being submerged by the Reformation. At the same time, both these subjects are so inextricably threaded through Geneva life that they will be dealt with, so to speak, *sur place* – i.e. as they occur in a particular context.

Notes

1. Weber, Johann (1750–93), known as John Webber. Son of Abraham Wäber, Swiss sculptor working in London. Official artist to Captain Cook on his last voyage to the South Seas.
2. Extract from a report to the government at Berne, in June 1818, from Albrecht von Haller, philosopher-poet and scientist: Fellow of the Royal Society in London.

CHAPTER *1*

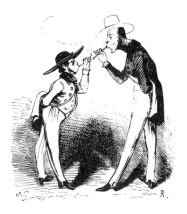

ON GENEVA

What impression did the small city of Geneva make on those who made their way there in the past as part of the Grand Tour? Writing in 1643 John Evelyn, on a brief and not entirely successful visit to Geneva, records in his diary:

> . . . a strong well-fortified city, part of it built on a rising ground. The houses are not despicable, but the high pent-houses, (for I can hardly call them cloisters, being all of wood) through which the people pass dry and in the shade, winter and summer, exceedingly deform the fronts of the buildings. Here are abundance of book-sellers; but their books are of ill impressions; these, with watches (of which store are made here), crystal, and excellent screwed guns, are the staple commodities. All provisions are good and cheap.[1]

Evelyn was a man who clearly had far more than his share of gifts, and he was unceasingly active in a whole variety of public offices throughout a long life. 'His manners we may presume to have been most agreeable: for his company was sought by the greatest men, not merely by inviting him to their own tables, but by their repeated visits to him at his own house', and, above all, William Bray, editor of his diary, tells us that he was astonishingly liberal and broadminded – managing to be personally attached to Charles I and James II, while at the same time having many

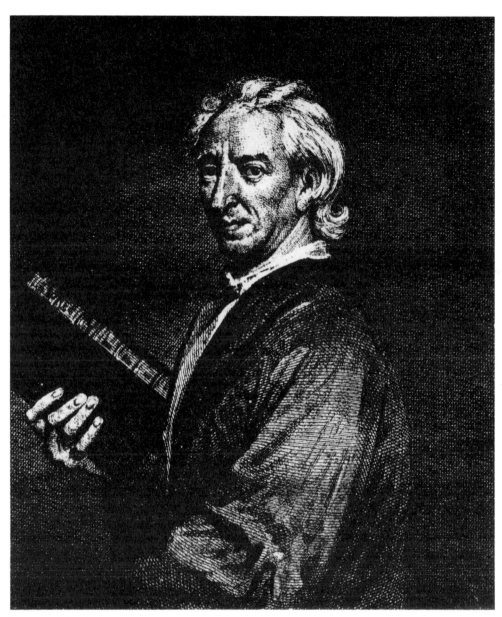

Portrait of John Evelyn,
probably by Kneller,
frontispiece to William
Bray's *Memoirs of John
Evelyn*, 1827

friends in Cromwell's entourage. Bray recounts that he set out
intending to join King Charles I at the Battle of Brentford,

> but subsequently desisting when the result of that battle
> became known, on the ground that his brother's as well as his
> own estate were so near London as to be fully in the power of
> the Parliament, and that their continued adherence would
> have been certain ruin to themselves without any advantage
> to His Majesty. In this dangerous conjuncture he asked and
> obtained the King's leave to travel.

This extended tour (1643–47) led Evelyn through France and
Italy, and thence to Switzerland, through the Simplon Pass.
Evelyn's travelling companion, Captain Wray, had with him his
water-spaniel, and at the top of the pass they were mobbed by an
angry crowd of villagers, who swore the dog had killed one of
their goats. Mass was about to be held in the little church, and the
party were held prisoner for its duration – being forced, later, to
pay a considerable fine. They were glad to escape and proceeded
down the mountain towards Brig in thick snow, having at one
point to dig out the pack-horse when it fell into a snow-drift.
     Continuing through the Valais, they were received with unu-
sual courtesy, both in Sion and then by the governor of St
Maurice. They went on to spend the night in Bouveret, where
they found the inn overfull with guests. Here Evelyn, who was
exhausted with a splitting headache, made the mistake of insisting
that the landlady turn her daughter out of bed for him.

> I went immediately into it whilst it was yet warm, being so
> heavy with pain and drowsiness that I would not stay to have
> the sheets changed; but I shortly paid dearly for my
> impatience, falling sick of the small-pox so soon as I came to
> Geneva, for by the smell of frankincense and the tale the
> good woman told me of her daughter having had an ague, I
> afterwards concluded she had been newly recovered of the
> small-pox.
>   I went with my company, the next day, hiring a bark to
> carry us over the lake; and indeed sick as I was, the weather
> was so serene never had travellers a sweeter passage . . . All
> this while, I held up tolerably, and the next morning, [in
> Geneva] having a letter for Signor John Diodati, the famous
> Italian minister and translator of the Holy Bible into that
> language, I went to his house and had a great deal of

discourse with that learned person. . . . After dinner, came one Monsieur Saladine, with his little pupil, the Earl of Caernarvon, to visit us, offering to carry us to the principal places of the town; but, being now no more able to hold up my head, I was constrained to keep my chamber, imagining that my very eyes would have dropped out . . . I was attended by a vigilant Swiss matron, whose monstrous throat, when I sometimes awaked out of unquiet slumbers, would affright me . . .

After sixteen days he recovered sufficiently to dine with Monsieur Saladine and, 'in the afternoon, went across the water on the side of the lake, and took a lodging that stood exceedingly pleasant . . . for the better airing, but I stayed only one night, having no company there, save my pipe . . .'

Evelyn then returned to Geneva, where he supped with Monsieur Saladine, and went to hear Dr Diodati

preach in French, and after the French mode, in a gown with a cape, and his hat on. The Church Government is severely Presbyterian, after the discipline of Calvin and Beza, who set it up, but nothing so rigid as either our Scots or English sectaries of that denomination. In the afternoon, M. Morice, a most learned young person and excellent poet, chief Professor of the University, preached at St Peter's, a spacious Gothic fabric. This was heretofore a cathedral and a reverend pile.

Later that day, Evelyn

. . . went to see the young townsmen exercise in Mars Field, where the prizes were pewter-plates and dishes; 'tis said that some have gained competent estates by what they have thus won. They were most accurate at the long-bow and musket, rarely missing the smallest mark. I was as busy with the carbine I brought from Brescia, as any of them. After dinner, Mr Morice led us to the college, a fair structure. They showed us a very ancient Bible, of about 300 years old, in the vulgar French . . .

The next day, Evelyn and his travelling companion, Captain Wray, prepared to continue their journey to Lyons. Before leaving Geneva Evelyn commented:

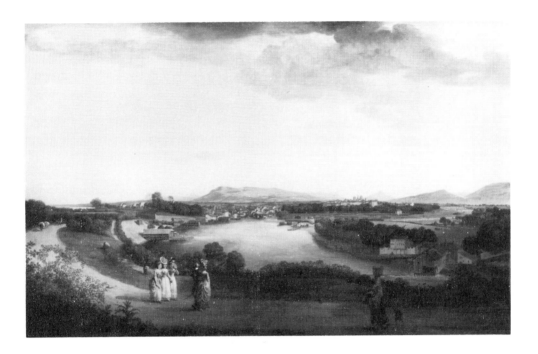

. . . This town is not much celebrated for beautiful women for, even at this distance from the Alps, the gentlewomen have something full throats, but our Captain Wray . . . fell so mightily in love with one of M. Saladine's daughters that, with much persuasion, he could not be prevailed on to think of his journey into France, the season now coming on extremely hot.

Geneva seen from the heights of Saint Jean, by Simon Malgo, 1778 (*Collection Musée d'art et d'histoire, Geneva*)

More than forty years later, Gilbert Burnet (1643–1715) spent several months in Geneva. Burnet – later to become Bishop of Salisbury – was an acknowledged champion of religious liberty and the historian of the English Reformation. He was of distinguished Scottish descent and apparently a delightful man:

. . . As a Friend, his conversation was always either useful or pleasant. He delivered himself with an Openness that shew'd he had no Reserves unworthy of a Minister or a Christian, and as none had it more in his Power to entertain a Companion, so his general Affability gave Access to Persons of lower Rank, and different Opinions.

As a Protestant, he had an early Reputation in the Reign of King Charles II, when *The Mystery of Iniquity was working fast*. Then he published his Noble 'History of the Reformation' . . . A sermon that he preached at the Rollo, in which he publish'd the Curses that King James I entail'd upon all his Posterity that ever turn'd Papist, set the Fury of the Court against him. Then he fled into Holland, and foreign Countries, and by the observations he made in his *Travels*, shew'd that the whole world could be a Library to him . . .[2]

Macaulay, in Chapter VII of his *History of England*, gives us a much-enlarged picture of Burnet.

. . . His high animal spirits, his boastfulness, his undissembled vanity, his propensity to blunder, his provoking indiscretion, his unabashed audacity, afforded inexhaustible subjects of ridicule to the Tories. Nor did his enemies omit to compliment him, sometimes with more pleasantry than delicacy, on the breadth of his shoulders, the thickness of calves, and his success in matrimonial projects on amorous and opulent widows. Yet, Burnet, though open in many respects to ridicule, and even to serious censure, was no contemptible man. His parts were quick, his industry unwearied, his reading various and most extensive. He was at once a historian, an antiquary, a theologian, a preacher, a pamphleteer, a debater, and an active political leader; and in every one of these characters he made himself conspicuous among able competitors. . . . A writer, whose voluminous works, in several branches of literature, find numerous readers 130 years after his death, may have had great faults, but must also have had great merits: and Burnet had great merits, a fertile and vigorous mind, a style, far indeed removed from faultless purity, but generally clear, often lively, and sometimes rising to solemn and fervid eloquence. In the pulpit the effect of his discourses, which were delivered without any note, was heightened by a noble figure and by pathetic action. He was often interrupted by the deep hum of his audience. . . . In his moral character, as in his intellect, great blemishes were more than compensated by great excellence. Though often misled by prejudice and passion, he was emphatically an honest man . . . His nature was kind, generous, grateful, forgiving. His religious zeal, though steady and ardent, was in general restrained by

humanity, and by a respect for the rights of conscience.
Strongly attached to what he regarded as the spirit of
Christianity, he looked with indifference on rites, names,
and forms of ecclesiastical polity, and was by no means
disposed to be severe even on infidels and heretics whose
lives were pure, and whose errors appeared to be the effect
rather of some perversion of the understanding than of the
depravity of the heart. But, like many other good men of that
age, he regarded the case of the Church of Rome as an
exception to all ordinary rules.

In *Some Letters, containing an Account of what seem'd most
remarkable in travelling thro' Switzerland, Italy, Some Parts of
Germany, Etc. in the Years 1685 and 1686*, Burnet describes how
he reached Geneva, by way of Paris, Lyons and Chambery. (He
must have arrived at about the moment of the Revocation of the
Edict of Nantes.)

. . . As I came all the way from *Paris* to *Lyons*, I was amazed
to see so much Misery as appear'd, not only in Villages, but
even in big Towns, where all the Marks of an extreme
Poverty shew'd themselves both in the Buildings, the
Cloaths, and almost in the Looks of the Inhabitants. And a
general Dispeopling in all the Towns, was a very visible
Effect of the Hardships under which they lay.

His description of Geneva is as lengthy as it is meticulous.

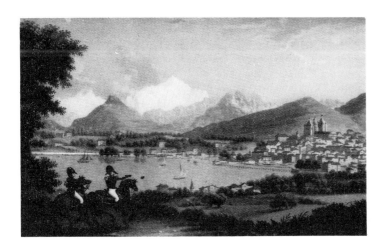

Gold musical snuff-box,
enamelled by J.-L.
Richter with a view of
Geneva and the Lake,
presentation-gift, 1815
(*Collection Musée d'art
et d'histoire, Geneva*)

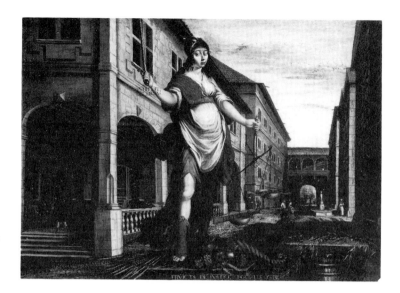

Allegorical painting, said to be of 'Justice', by Samuel de Raméru, *c*. 1650 (*Collection Musée d'art et d'histoire, Geneva*)

. . . Geneva is too well-known to be much insisted on. It is a little State; but it has so many good Constitutions in it, that the greatest may justly learn of it. The Chamber of the Corn has always two Years Provision for the City in Store, and forces none but the bakers to buy of it at a taxed Price; and so it is both necessary against any Extremities under which the State may fall, and is likewise of great Advantage; for it gives a good yearly Income, that has help'd the State to pay near a Million of Debts contracted during the Wars: And the Citizens are not oppress'd by it; for every Inhabitant may buy his own Corn as he pleases, only publick Houses must buy from the Chamber. And if one will compare the Faith of *Rome* and *Geneva* together by this Particular, he would be forced to prefer the latter: For if *good Works* are a strong Presumption, if not a sure Indication of a *good Faith*, then *Justice*, being a good Work of the first Form, Geneva will certainly carry it.

At *Rome* the Pope buys in all the Corn of the Patrimony; for none of the Landlords can sell it either to Merchants or Bakers. He buys it at five Crowns their Measure, and even that is slowly and ill paid; so that there was eight hundred thousand Crowns owing upon that Score when I was at *Rome*. . . . [And much more to Rome's detriment] . . .

Whereas in *Geneva*, the Measure by which they buy and sell
is the same; and the Gain is so inconsiderable, that it is very
little beyond the common Market-Price: So that upon the
whole matter the Chamber of Corn is but the Merchant to
the State. But if the Publick makes a moderate Gain by the
Corn, that and all the other Revenues of this small Common-
wealth are so well employ'd that there is no Cause of
Complaint given in the Administration of the publick Purse,
which with the Advantages that arise out of the Chamber of
the Corn is about an hundred thousand Crowns Revenue.
But there is much to go out of this: Three hundred Soldiers
are paid, an Arsenal is maintain'd, that in Proportion to the
State is the greatest in the World, for it contains Arms for
more Men than are in the State:

There is a great Number of Ministers and Professors, in all
twenty four, paid out of it, besides all the publick Charges
and Offices of the Government. Every one of the lesser
Council of twenty five having an hundred Crowns, and every
Syndic having two hundred Crowns Pension; and, after all
this, come the accidental Charges of the Deputies, that they
are obliged to send often to *Paris*, to *Savoy*, and to
Switzerland; so that it is very apparent no Man can enrich
himself at the Cost of the Publick. And the Appointments of
the *Little Council* are a very Recompence for the great
Attendance that they are obliged to give the Publick, which
is commonly four or five Hours a Day. The Salary for the
Professors and Ministers is indeed small, not above two
hundred Crowns; but to balance this (which was a more
competent Provision, when it was first set off a hundred and
fifty Years ago, the Price of all Things, and the Way of
Living being now much heighten'd) those Employments are
here held in their due Reputation; and the richest Citizens in
the Town breed up their Children so as to qualify them for
those Places. And a Minister that is suitable to his Character,
is thought so good a Match, that generally they have such
Estates either by Succession or Marriage, as support them
suitably to the Rank they hold. And in *Geneva* there is so
great a Regulation upon Expenses of all Sorts that a small
Sum goes a great way. It is a surprising thing to see so much
Learning as one finds in *Geneva*, not only among those
whose Profession obliges them to study, but among the
Magistrate and Citizens; And if there are not many Men of
the first Form of Learning among them, yet almost every-

body here has a good Tincture of a learned Education, insomuch that they are Masters of the *Latin*, they know History and the Controversies of Religion, and are generally Men of good Sense.

There is a universal Civility, not only towards Strangers, but towards one another, that reigns all the Town over, and leans to an Excess: So that in them one sees a Mixture of a *French* Openness, and an *Italian* Exactness; there is indeed a little too much of the last.

Burnet continues his detailed picture of the Geneva of his day:

The publick Justice of the City is quick and good, and is more commended than the private Justice of those that deal in Trade: A want of Sincerity is much lamented by those that know the Town well. There is no publick Lewdness tolerated, and the Disorders of that sort are managed with great Address. And notwithstanding their Neighbourhood to the Switzers, Drinking is very little known among them.

And he goes on to express strong approval of the way in which they buy and sell 'Estates', under the control of the government:

This Government is the same both in *Geneva* and in most of the Cantons. The Sovereignty lies in the *Council of Two Hundred*: and this Council chooses out of its Number twenty five, who are *the lesser Council*; and the Censure of the *Twenty five* belongs to the *Great Council*. They are chosen by a sort of Ballot, so that it is not known for whom they give their Votes; which is an effectual Method to suppress Factions and Resentments, since in a Competition no man can know who voted for him or against him: Yet the Election is not so carried, but that the whole Town is in a Intrigue concerning it: For since the being of the *Little Council* leads one to the *Sindicate*, which is the chief Honour of the State, this Dignity is courted here with as active and solicitous an Ambition as appears elsewhere for greater matters. The *Two Hundred* are chosen and censured by the *Twenty Five*; so that these two Councils, which are both for Life, are Checks one upon another: The Magistracy is in the one, and Sovereignty in the other . . .

[There is] a further Council, consisting of those of the two hundred that have born Offices, such as Auditors, Attorney

Generals . . . This Court has no Authority, but is call'd together by the *Twenty Five*, when any extraordinary Occasion makes it advisable for them to call for a more general Concurrence in the Resolutions that they are about to form . . . The whole Body of the Burgesses choose the Syndics the first Sunday of the Year . . . The Difference between the Burgesses and Citizens is, that the former Degree may be bought, or given to Strangers, and they are capable to be of the *Two Hundred*; but none is a Citizen, but he that is the Son of a Burgess, and that is born within the Town.

Gilbert Burnet ends

I need say no more of the Constitution of this little Republick. Its chief Support is in the firm Alliance that has stood now so long between it and the Cantons of *Berne* and *Zurich*; and it is so visibly the Interest of all Switzerland to preserve it, as the Key by which it may be all laid open, that if the Cantons had not forgotten their Interest so palpably, in suffering the *French* to become Masters of the *Franche Comte*, one would think that they would not be capable of suffering *Geneva* to be touch'd: For all that can be done in fortifying the Town can signify no more, than to put it in a Case to resist a Surprize or Scalade; since if a Royal Army comes against it to besiege it in Form, it is certain, that unless the *Switzers* come down with a Force able to raise the Siege, those within will be able to make but a very short Resistance.

Gilbert Burnet left Geneva at the end of August 1685 and continued his journey through Switzerland to Italy. He returned in December and passed the winter there. This jolly, human prelate-to-be, with his lack of tact and 'animal spirits', was later to render his country a unique service – in bringing about a reconciliation between William of Orange and his wife Mary. In the meantime, he was back in a place which he clearly found to his taste.

. . . I pass the Winter at *Geneva* with more Satisfaction than I had thought it was possible for me to have found anywhere out of England; tho' that received great Allays from the most lamentable Stories that we had every day from France; but *there is a Sorrow by which the Heart is made better*. I ought to make the most publick Acknowledgements possible for the

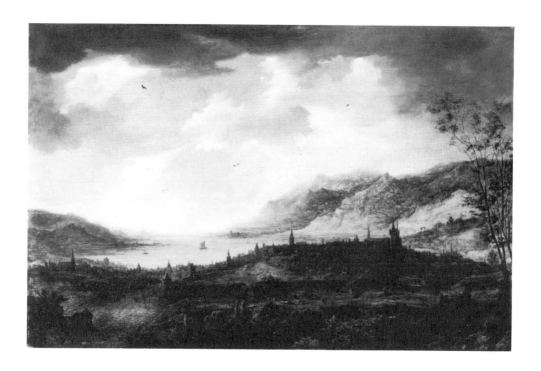

View of Geneva at the beginning of the seventeenth century, by José Momper (*Collection Musée d'art et d'histoire, Geneva*)

extraordinary Civilities that I met with in my own particular; but that is too low a Subject to entertain you with. That which pleased me most was of a more publick Nature. Before I left *Geneva* the Number of the *English* there was such, that I found we could make a small Congregation, for we were twelve or fourteen; so I addressed myself to the Council of *Twenty Five*, for Liberty to have our own Worship in our own Language, according to the *English* Liturgy. This was immediately granted in so obliging a manner, that as there was not one Person that made any Exception to it, so they sent one of their Body to me, to let me know, that in case our Number should grow to be so great that it were fit for us to assemble in a Church, they would grant us one which had been done in Queen Mary's Reign; but till then, we might hold our Assemblies as we thought fit. So after that time, during the rest of my Stay there, we had every *Sunday* our Devotions according to the Common Prayer Morning and Evening; and at the Evening-Prayer I preach'd in a Room that was indeed too large for our small Company: But there being a considerable Number in *Geneva* that understand

English, and in particular some of the Professors and
Ministers, we had a great many Strangers that met with us;
and the last *Sunday* I gave the Sacrament according to the
Way of the Church of *England*; and upon this Occasion I
found a general Joy in the Town for this, that I had given
them an Opportunity of expressing the Respect they had for
our Church. And as in their publick Prayers they always
pray'd for the Churches of *Great Britain*, as well as for the
King, so in private Discourse they shewed all possible
Esteem for our Constitutions; and they spoke of the unhappy
Divisions among us, and of the Separation that was made
from us upon the account of our Government and Cere-
monies, with great Regret and Dislike. I shall name to you
only two of their Professors, that, as they are Men of great
Distinction, so they were the Persons with whom I conver-
sed the most: The one is Mr *Turretin*, a Man of great
Learning, that by his indefatigable Study and Labour has
much worn out and wasted his Strength, amidst all the
Affluence of a great Plenty of Fortune to which he was born;
one discerns in him all the Modesty of an humble and
mortified Temper, and of an active and fervent Charity,
proportioned to his Abundance, or rather beyond it; and
there is in him such a melting Zeal for Religion, as the
present Conjuncture calls for, with all the Seriousness of
Piety and Devotion, which shews itself both in private
Conversation and in his most edifying Sermons, by which he
enters deep into the Consciences of his Hearers. The other is
Mr Tronchin, a Man of a strong head, and of a clear and
correct Judgement, who has all his Thoughts well digested:
His Conversation has an engaging Charm in it, that cannot
be resisted: He is a Man of extraordinary Virtue, and of a
Readiness to oblige and serve all Persons, that has scarce any
Measures: His Sermons have a Sublimity in them that
strikes the Hearer, as well as it edifies him; his Thoughts are
noble, and his Eloquence is masculine and exact, and has all
the Majesty of the Chair in it, tempered with all the
Softeness of Persuasion; so that he not only convinces his
Hearers, but subdues them, and triumphs over them. In
such Company it was no wonder if Time seemed to go off too
fast, so that I left *Geneva* with a Concern that I could not
have felt in leaving any Place out of the Isle of *Britain*.

This, then, was a distinguished cleric's view of the Geneva

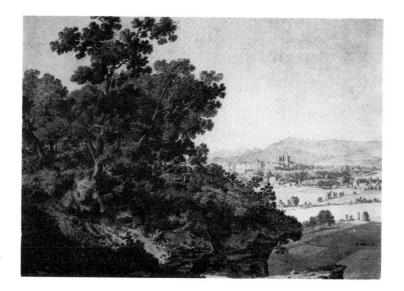

Geneva seen from the
Bois de la Bâtie, by
Jean-Antoine Link
(*Collection Musée d'art
et d'histoire, Geneva*)

which was attracting increasing numbers of Englishmen in the
second half of the seventeenth century.

An unpublished *mémoire* by Monsieur Edouard Pictet, *The
English In Geneva*, which won him the Prix Harvey in 1938,
gives some insight into Anglo-Genevese relations, in the context
of mid- and late-seventeenth-century European politics.

> . . . In 1674, the English living in Geneva were very shaken
> by the kidnapping of one of their group, the 'Chevalier
> d'Harvey' – an English Milord who was hunting at *La
> Servette*.[3] The affair which made a great impression at the
> time was very lively. It ended with the arrest of Pierre and
> Isaac Baudichon of the Maison Neuve, who had in fact let
> their victim escape 'in the place of the Redheads' (Lieu des
> Rousses). They sent a search-party accompanied by a dele-
> gate to net the prisoners who did not wait for the arrival of
> justice, and made their escape. The story ended with the
> condemnation of the guilty parties for contempt of court –
> one to have his head cut off, the other to be banished for life.

Pictet also refers to a letter from Pierre Mussard (1626–81), an
étudiant at Geneva and minister in 1654, who at the end of his life
was a pastor in London. In this letter addressed to his wife, he

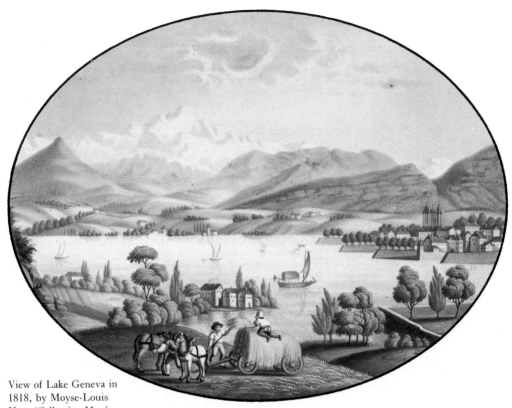

View of Lake Geneva in
1818, by Moyse-Louis
Hess (*Collection Musée
d'art et d'histoire,
Geneva*)

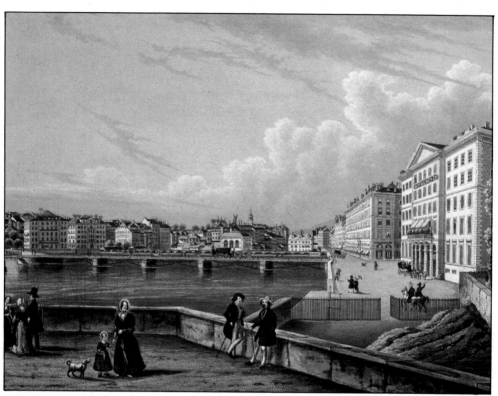

View from the Quai des
Bergues in 1845, by
Dickenman
(*Photograph: Nicolas
Bouvier*)

mentions that Charles II had announced publicly, 'Those in Geneva are giving safe hiding to the murderers of the King my father; to such an extent that they have given them guards; are those the instructions of Calvin . . . ?'

In his *mémoire* Pictet gives the following account of the situation in which Geneva found itself in 1689:

. . . In 1689 Geneva found itself in considerable danger – terrified in fact of offending both France and Britain. On November 4th, Iberville, French Ambassador [Resident] to Geneva, declared clearly that 'he had received orders from the King that in the event of his learning of the arrival of the Resident of England, he would remove himself *sans congé*, and that he would leave it to the prudence of those who governed [Geneva] to reflect on the consequences that his departure could bring.[4]

Pictet continued:

Chouet, professor of philosophy and member of the Syndic 1699, was instructed to write to Gilbert Burnet, now Bishop of Salisbury, and a staunch supporter of William of Orange. It was equally arranged that the *Syndic de la Rive* would write to M. Escher, *bourgmestre* of Zurich, to ask him to confer with Mr Thomas Coxe (representative of the English Court to the Swiss cantons) 'to make him understand our true interests.'

. . . It is certain, Milord, that the first news we had of this *envoi* [i.e. the impending arrival of William II's *envoyé*, Des Marais] – filled with universal iodine all our People as well as the Magistrate; [who] have considered it as a sign of the affection with which this incomparable Prince honours us . . . But Monsieur the Resident of France does not receive it as we do; he published first that in the state in which affairs were, there was complete incompatibility between a resident of England and himself . . . He renews all his threats, and adds that he has been ordered to remove himself even *sans prendre congé*, when he learns that Monsieur Des Marais is on his way.

In other words, the Council was now quite desperate to postpone the arrival of England's ambassador.

On 16 December the news erupted that Des Marais was at St

Gall. On 22 December Herwarth was in Geneva. His last instructions from London had been:

> . . . from the King to Mr Philibert d'Herwarth. Instruction vor our trusty and well-beloved Philibert d'Herwarth whom Ve have appointed to reside in the quality of our Envoyé with the Republic of Geneva . . . You shall forth with . . . repair to Geneva and being arrived there demand an Audience of the Senate at which you shall . . . particularly assure them that we being bound with them in one common type of Religion shall always have a peculiar regard to what concerns their welfare and Interest.

On 23 October, when Herwarth was *en route*, he received further instructions:

> Considering the great danger which threatens the city of Geneva of being surprised by the French or forced to submit to them. We think it necessary you should make all haste you possibly can thither. On your way thither you shall with all the privacy you can call upon Thomas Coxe Esqur.,[5] our Envoyé Entraordinary with the Cantons of Switzerland.

Des Marais, as we have seen, had arrived in Geneva on 22 December, but only on 2 January did he declare himself. The Council, at its wit's end to know what to do, kept him waiting sixteen days before acknowledging his credentials. Eventually he expressed in strongest terms his displeasure and withdrew to Berne. The French, of course, then moved in.

As the eighteenth century unrolled, French influence in Geneva alternated with ever-closer ties with England. The Genevan banking system established itself early in the century and there was brisk buying on the part of Genevan traders on the English market, as well as extensive investment in English government stock. More and more Genevans, together with Swiss from other cantons, made their way to London – establishing a pattern for the future.

The English, in their turn and according to their interests, were becoming thoroughly familiar with the road to Geneva. Thomas Pennant (1726–96), natural scientist of distinction, author of *British Zoology*, and immortalised in his correspondence with the naturalist Gilbert White in *The Natural History of*

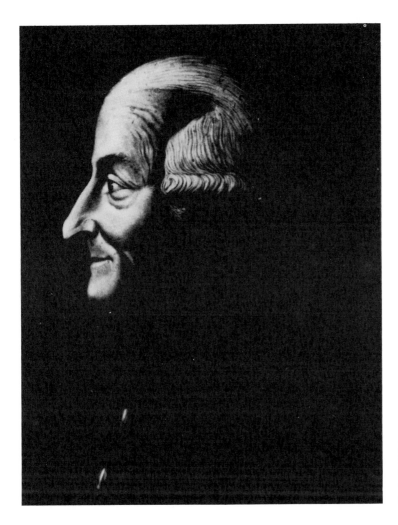

Jean-André de Luc
(1727–1817), geologist
and meteorologist
(*Collection Musée d'art
et d'histoire, Geneva*)

Selborne, came to Geneva in 1765. Meticulous in all he did, he seems hardly to have been the life and soul of any party, but Boswell reports that Dr Johnson observed in his defence, 'he's a Whig, sir; a sad dog. But he's the best traveller I ever read; he observes more things than anyone else does.'

Pennant decided to make a Continental tour in order to visit fellow-scientists.[6] After spending some time with the comte de Buffon in Paris, he notes laconically in his diary:

. . . Took the usual route to Lyon . . . ; and, on arrival in

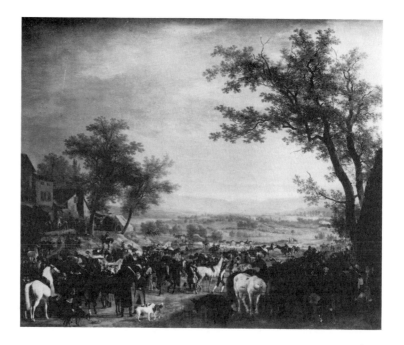

The Horse-market at Gaillard by James Agasse, end of the seventeenth century, (the scenery was painted by A. W. Töpffer) (*Collection Musée d'art et d'histoire, Geneva*)

Geneva . . . I entered the city through the Porte Neuve and retired to a good Inn, where I was confined this evening and the following day with a severe cold.

May 3rd Waited on Messieurs de Luc,[7] the Father and two Sons, who during my stay paid me every attention. I shall often have occasion to speak of the considerable light I received from the labor of John Andrew, the Younger [recte: elder] son, vz. who has immortalised himself by his improvements of the Barometer, and by his accurate application of that instrument for the measurement of the heights of mountains.

There follows a highly detailed account of Geneva, showing that Pennant was indeed a man of meticulous observation.

. . . The situation [of Geneva] is admirable, – bounded on the north by the Lake, on the west by the Rhone, and on the south and east by the rich plains watered by the Arve. The views from several parts are unparalleled for grandeur and beauty . . .

And he instances

Le Bastion or La Promenade, a beautiful garden planted
with trees and shrubs . . . All amusements which conduce to
corrupt the morals are banished from the city. Its legislature
planned this innocent elegance in order to re-create the
citizens in their leisure hours. Above this is a fine walk under
the shade of Horse Chestnuts now in full bloom, called *La
Treille*. The prospect from this beautiful terrace is very fine
. . . La Maison de Ville or Town House stands immediately
above this walk. The winding staircase is very singular,
being without steps and paved from bottom to top, so that it
may be readily ascended on horse-back.

Two inscriptions on brass plates fixed at the entrance
remind the citizens of the signal events of their two great
deliverances: the one of their freedom from the papal power
in 1535, the other of their escape from slavery to the house of
Savoy by the detection of the infamous attempt made to
surprise the city in 1602. In the arsenal, which is adjacent to
the town house, are preserved numbers of the instruments
employed by the Savoyards . . . and the very petard ready
charged which was fastened to one of the gates to burst it
open; when the gunner was killed before it could be dischar-
ged. This perfidious plan was put in execution at midnight of
November 12th Old style. The forces of Savoy were assembled in the neighbourhood, and those allotted for the
Escalade in the *plein palais*, where they were confessed and
absolved by a Scotch Jesuit who furnished with little tickets,
inscribed with texts of holy writ, the three hundred to whom
this desperate part of the enterprise was assigned, assuring
them that by virtue of those 'who fell below, should meet the
prize above'.

About two hundred got into the city; the alarm was given;
and by the gallant behaviour of the inhabitants the assailants
were partly slain, partly forced to leap over the walls to their
expecting confederates on the outside, who were waiting to
seize their prey on the bursting of the city gates to which the
petard was applied. Seventeen citizens died in defence of
their country, and were honourably interred. Thirteen of the
enemy who were taken alive were next day hanged upon the
ramparts, being considered as common robbers who had
violated the laws of nations, unworthy of the treatment due

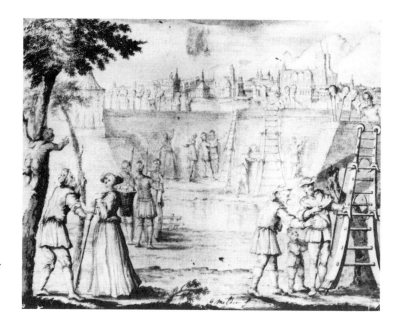

Geneva the day after
the *Escalade*, signed
'G. Milder 5', end of
the seventeenth century
(*Bibliothèque Publique
et Universitaire,
Geneva*)

to an open foe. Their heads and those of fifty four found slain
in the town were placed on stakes in rows on the walls facing
Savoy, as a mark of infamy for so nefarious an enterprise;
their bodies were denied burial, and flung with disgrace into
the Rhone . . .

It is interesting to note that throughout this spirited account of
the 'Escalade' no mention is made of Geneva's national heroine,
La Mère Royaume, who is said to have halted the initial vanguard
of Savoyards as they scaled the walls by pouring the red-hot
contents of a vast *marmotte* (cooking-pot) over them.

. . . The Church of St Peter, the cathedral of popish days,
stands a little higher on the loftiest part of the hill . . . It was
totally destroyed by fire on the 1st April 1430, excepting a
tower on the side of the lake. The church was not totally
rebuilt till 1510. The present building is adorned with a
modern portico in front, supported by four pillars of the
corinthian order. Iconoclastic fury in the year of the reformation has despoiled it of all ornament except the windows at
the east end which are of painted glass.
On the 5th May I attended divine service at this church,

and had opportunity of observing the simplicity of Calvinistic worship. Prayers began at nine, at which time all the city gates are shut and two of the officers called Auditeurs, attended by others, go round the town during sermon time to prevent people from going about, unless upon some very important occasions. A young clergyman first read the commandments out of the Pulpit. He then gave way to an elder divine, who, after a long prayer, published contracts of matrimony between several couples; a Psalm was given out and sung in the old English fashion, accompanied with the organ. He then made a short extemporary prayer, and repeated that of our Lord. A sermon followed, which lasted half an hour; after which was sung another Psalm. The minister repeated the creed, and concluded with a prayer for the whole state of mankind. At the beginning of the sermon he put on his hat, as did several of the congregation, who sit promiscuously. Strangers are allowed a seat to themselves.

The wise and peripatetic cleric, Archdeacon William Coxe (1747–1828), paid four visits to Switzerland in the latter half of the eighteenth century. Coxe was educated at Eton and ordained in 1771. After a brief curacy, he became tutor to the Duke of Marlborough's eldest son and two years later was made travelling tutor to the son of the Earl of Pembroke. He travelled widely in the mid-eighteenth century through Switzerland and parts of Russia; later, he made two further tours to the Continent, revisiting Switzerland on each occasion. A prolific and perceptive writer, he published *The Historical and Political State of Europe* in 1772, followed by *Sketches of the National Political and Civil State of Swisserland* in 1789. Like Burnet a hundred years earlier, Coxe is fascinated by the Genevan system of government and, like him, delighted at the educational opportunities available to all citizens:

To a man of letters Geneva is particularly interesting; learning is divested of pedantry, and philosophy united with a knowledge of the world; the pleasures of Society are mixed with the pursuits of literature, and elegance and urbanity give a zest to the profoundest disquisitions . . . Even the lower class of people are exceedingly well-informed, and there is perhaps no city in Europe where learning is more universally diffused.

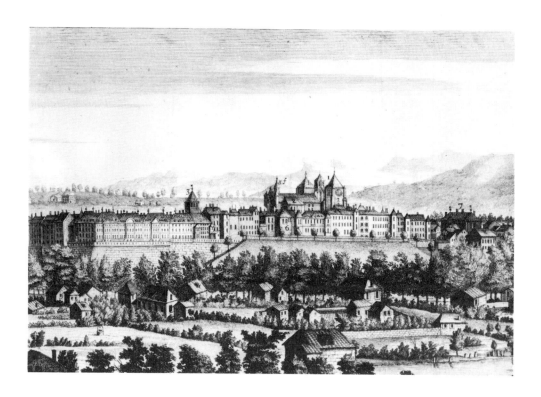

The Ramparts, Geneva,
late eighteenth century
(*Bibliothèque Publique
et Universitaire,
Geneva*)

John Moore[8] gives us a different, and more personal, description of the Geneva of the 1770s. Moore was a distinguished young Scottish physician chosen by the Duchess of Hamilton to be tutor to her son Douglas on a prolonged 'Grand Tour' of Europe. Tutor and pupil spent a considerable time in Geneva, and Moore writes easily:

> . . . The situation of Geneva is in many respects as happy as the heart of man could define, or his imagination conceive. The Rhône, rushing out of the noblest lake in Europe, flows through the middle of the city, which is encircled by fertile fields, cultivated by the industry, and adorned by the riches and taste, of the inhabitants.
>
> The long ridge of mountains called Mount Jura on the one side, with the Alps, the Glaciers of Savoy, and the snowy head of Mont Blanc on the other, serve as boundaries to the most charmingly variegated landscape that ever delighted the eye.
>
> With these advantages in point of situation, the citizens of

Geneva enjoy freedom untainted by licentiousness, and security unbought by the horrors of war.

The great number of men of letters, who either are natives of the place, or have chosen it for their residence, the decent manners, the easy circumstances, and humane dispositions of the Genevois in general, render this city and its environs a very desirable retreat for people of a philosophic turn of mind.

An education here is equally cheap and liberal, the citizens of Geneva of both sexes are remarkably well instructed. I do not imagine that any country in the world can produce an equal number of persons (taken without selection from all degrees and professions) with minds so much cultivated as the inhabitants of Geneva possess.

It is not uncommon to find mechanics in the intervals of their labour amusing themselves with the works of Locke, Montesquieu, Newton, and other productions of the same kind.

When I speak of the cheapness of a liberal education, I mean for the natives and citizens only; for strangers now find everything dear at Geneva. Wherever Englishmen resort, this is the case. If they do not find things dear, they soon make them so.

The democratical nature of their government inspires every citizen with an idea of his own importance: He perceives that no man in the republic can insult, or even neglect him, with impunity . . . As far as I can judge, a spirit of independency and freedom, tempered by sentiments of decency and the love of order, influence, in a most remarkable manner, the minds of the subjects of this happy republic.

Before I knew them, I had formed an opinion, that the people of this place were fanatical, gloomy-minded, and unsociable, as the puritans in England, and the presbyterians in Scotland were, during the civil wars, and the reigns of Charles II and his brother. In this, however, I find I had conceived a very erroneous notion.

There is not, I may venture to assert, a city in Europe where the minds of the people are less under the influence of superstition or fanatical enthusiasm than at Geneva.

The clergy of Geneva in general are men of sense, learning, and moderation, impressing upon the minds of their hearers the tenets of Christianity with all the graces of pulpit eloquence, and illustrating the efficacy of the doctrine by their conduct in life . . . There is one custom universal here, and, as far as I know, peculiar to this place: The parents form societies for their children at a very early period of their lives. These societies consist of ten, a dozen, or more children of the same sex, and nearly of the same age and situation in life. They assemble once a week in the houses of the different parents, who entertain the company by turns with tea, coffee, biscuits and fruit; and then leave the young assembly to the freedom of their own conversation.

This connection is strictly kept up through life, whatever alterations may take place in the situations or circumstances of the individuals. And although they should afterwards form new or preferable intimacies, they never entirely abandon this society; but to the latest period of their lives continue to pass a few evenings every year with the companions of their youth and their earliest friends.

The richer class of the citizens have country-houses adjacent to the town, where they pass one half of the year. These houses are all of them neat, and some of them splendid. One piece of magnificence they possess in greater perfection than the most superb villa of the greatest lord in any other part of the world can boast, I mean the prospect which almost all of them command – The gardens, and vineyards of the republic – the Pais de Vaux; – Geneva with its lake; – innumerable country-seats; – cattles, and little towns around the lake; – the vallies of Savoy, and the loftiest mountains of the Alps, all within one sweep of the eye.

Those whose fortunes or employments do not permit them to pass the summer in the country, make frequent parties of pleasure upon the lake, and dine and spend the evening at some of the villages in the environs, where they amuse themselves with music and dancing . . .

The mildness of the climate, the sublime beauties of the country, and the agreeable manners of the inhabitants, are not, in my opinion, the greatest attractions of this place.

Upon the same hill, in the neighbourhood of Geneva, three English families at present reside, whose society would render any country agreeable.

The house of Mr N— is a temple of hospitality, good humour, and friendship.

Near to him lives your acquaintance Mr U—. He perfectly answers your description, lively, sensible, and obliging; and, I imagine, happier than ever you saw him, having since that time drawn a great prize in the matrimonial lottery.

Their nearest neighbours are the family of Mr L—. This gentleman, his lady and children, form one of the most pleasing pictures of domestic felicity I ever beheld. He himself is a man of refined taste, a benevolent mind, and elegant manners.

These three families, who live in the greatest cordiality with the citizens of Geneva, their own countrymen, and one another, render the hill of Cologny the most delightful place perhaps at this moment in the world.

The English gentlemen, who reside in the town, often resort hither, and mix with parties of the best company in Geneva.

I am told, that our young countrymen never were on so friendly and sociable a footing with the citizens of this republic as at present, owing in a great degree to the conciliatory manners of these three families, and to the great popularity of an English nobleman, who has lived with his lady and son in this state for several years.

The nobleman and his family referred to by John Moore was clearly Philip, Lord Stanhope.[9] In his boyhood, as the young Lord Mahon, he was sent by his father, Charles Stanhope, to study French in Geneva. The Stanhopes were all active Whigs, and keen public servants. Philip's grandfather, James, was one of George I's principal private secretaries and they were connected with the Pitts. Later on, Philip, who had succeeded his father, returned to Geneva with his own family. He, his wife (née Hamilton), and two teenage sons, Philip and Charles, settled in Sécheron, where they remained for twelve years. Philip died at the age of seventeen. The Council of Geneva went to Sécheron to offer their condolences. Lord Stanhope, who from emotion and an inability to express himself in French (a failing which remained with him), gave the councillors a document in which he expressed not only his thanks but also the warmest feelings in general concerning the Council. Thereafter, the Stanhopes were given permission to put up an inscription near their son's grave: an unusual privilege for foreigners in Geneva.

The Stanhopes showed their attachment to Geneva in many practical ways, not least by generous donations to the city's hospital, and were on the warmest terms with the authorities. Their young son, Charles (Lord Mahon), was evidently excep-

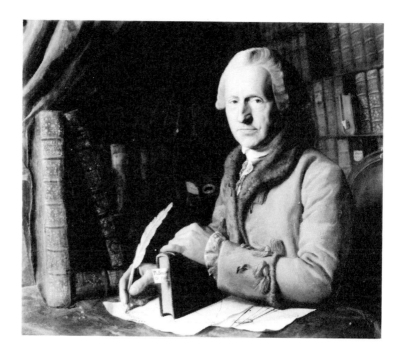

Lord Stanhope
(previously Lord
Mahon) (*Bibliothèque
Publique et
Universitaire, Geneva*)

tionally gifted in 'mechanical sciences', and became an outstanding
student. He was also very fond of sport, and in 1771, as a guest at
a dinner given by the Archery Society, he took part in their
annual competition. Although a complete novice, he carried off
first prize, thus earning himself the title of 'Commander of
Archery'. The next day the Geneva Council made him a bourgeois of the city, as no foreigner was allowed to become Commander unless he were either a bourgeois or a citizen. At the same
time, mindful of the excellent relations existing between Geneva
and Charles's father, the Council conferred the same honour on
Lord Stanhope. Charles was proclaimed Commander and
accompanied home by all the 'officers, chevaliers and tambours',
the latter playing the march of the [Archery] Exercise. This
considerable *cortège* was received with the greatest courtesy by
his parents.

As a result of all this mutual goodwill, the young Lord Mahon
asked and obtained permission to give, in his turn and at his own
expense, a 'fête' at Pré l'Evêque, home of the Society. Unfortunately, this event was rained out, and so he arranged that the
first half of the programme, a dinner for some three hundred
people, would take place at the Hôtel du Village.

A week later, the deferred fête took place at Pré l'Evèque and a week after that, the new Commander was 'installed' according to custom. The whole exercise terminated with a party on the lake eight months afterwards.

Two years later, in August 1773, when Lord Mahon was relinquishing his role of Commander, he made a speech in which he stressed the efforts he had made – 'being Genevois' – to give amusement to his co-citizens. After complimenting his officers on their zeal and intelligence, he finished:

> . . . I was brought up in Geneva, and I love this town as my second country; and I will always love it as long as virtue and liberty reign within these walls; and God willing, this will be for ever. Although I cease today to be Commander of Archery, I will never forget that I have filled this post, or that I have the good fortune to be counted amongst the *Bourgeois* of this Republic.

The Stanhopes left Geneva in an atmosphere of mutual esteem and regret that was practically euphoric and, on their return to London, Charles assumed his place amongst the Liberals in Parliament. In 1782, however, he had occasion to write in the strongest terms to the first councillor of Geneva, Buffe, on the subject of Ami Melly, the leader of a group of Genevois who had emigrated to Ireland following the political strife in Geneva in 1782. Melly had taken English nationality, which secured him British protection when Geneva attempted to take proceedings against him. Lord Mahon expressed his outrage at such an abuse of liberty on the part of the Geneva Council, concluding, 'As far as I am concerned, the only favour I ask the Council is to have my name removed from the roll of *Bourgeois* of your Republic.'

The Council quite simply decided to ignore this communication. After the revolution of 1792 reached Geneva, the new régime wrote in May 1794 to Citizen Stanhope, inviting him to regard himself as reinstated within the rights of the city of Geneva. Stanhope replied in March 1795, writing from Chevening House, near Sevenoaks, Kent. He explained that the law no longer allowed him to accept the title of 'Citizen' which they had given him the honour of renewing – underlining that his refusal had nothing whatever to do with his original renunciation of the rights of Bourgeois.

The Stanhope era in Geneva must have been an unusually golden one. How easy it is to sense the warmth and enthusiasm

generated by Charles Mahon's victory and the ensuing cele-
brations to mark the new Commander of Archery's installation.
As for John Moore's description of the three English families
'living on the hill' at Cologny, the picture presented is one of
uncluttered harmony between English and Genevese.

Notes

1. *Diary and correspondence of John Evelyn Esq., FRS,* edited by
   William Bray, 1827.
2. *A Character of the Rt. Reverend Father-in-God, Gilbert [Burnet],
   Lord Bishop of Sarum,* printed for J. Roberts, near the Oxford-
   Arms, in Warwick-Lane, 1715.
3. Edward D'Ervil de Montaigu, chevalier d'Harvey.
4. The Council of Geneva had long been negotiating with William
   of Orange (before, in fact, his actual ascent to the throne of
   England) for help in opposing the French. It was as a result of
   these negotiations that William decided to send Mr Philibert
   d'Herwarth Des Marais as his envoye in Geneva. The Resident
   of France was well aware of the situation.
5. Thomas Coxe, envoye to the Swiss Confederation.
6. *Tour on the Continent,* Thomas Pennant, 1765. Edited with
   notes by G.R. de Beer, 1945.
7. Jacques-Francois de Luc, 1698–1782, watch-maker; Jean-Andre
   de Luc, 1727–1817, Fellow of the Royal Society 10 June 1773,
   geologist and meteorologist; and Guillaume-Antoine de Luc,
   1729–1812, conchologist.
8. *A View of Society and Manners in France, Switzerland and
   Germany, with anecdotes relating to some eminent characters,*
   John Moore, London, Straham and Cadell, 1779.
9. *L'Ancienne Geneve,* Louis Dufour-Vernes, 1909.

CHAPTER 2

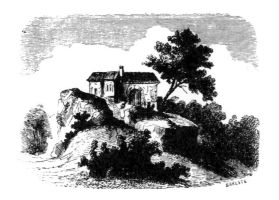

THE

SAGE OF FERNEY

One of the great attractions offered by Geneva in the last decades of the eighteenth century was undoubtedly the proximity of the 'Sage of Ferney'. Voltaire, on the run from France, took refuge in Geneva, where the authorities gave him a cautious welcome. Before long he acquired Les Délices, a small property at Ferney, about four miles from Geneva in the Pays de Gex. This was actually on French soil, but several Swiss families lived in the surrounding villages. In Pennant's words, 'he found an ancient Chateau on the Estate, which he pulled down, and built a very moderate house, in its room.' A private theatre was added and here the old reprobate settled down to perpetuate the Voltaire legend.

This was a moment when Rousseau's 'happy savage' philosophy largely dominated Europe's intellectual scene. Provocative as it was, his theme of an ideal society with the emphasis on Man's need to return to natural simplicity, without society's corruptive culture, was widely discussed in European capitals, and not least in his native Geneva. Boswell, coming from Germany on his Grand Tour in 1764, called on Rousseau at Môtiers. The visit was an unusual success, and in a state of euphoria he then continued to Geneva, where he arrived on Saturday 22 December. That night he wrote in his diary:

. . . I had a good day's drive to Geneva [from Lausanne]. Yesterday had slept only two hours. Set out a little after four,

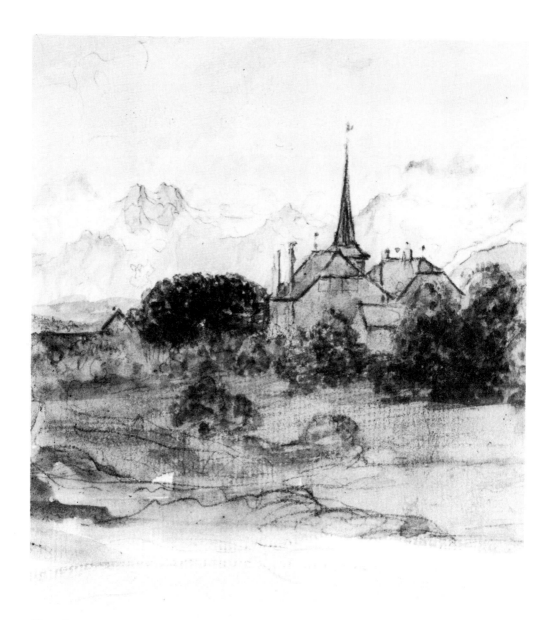

View of a village with a
church spire, against a
background of high
peaks, by Huber the
Elder (*Collection Musée
d'art et d'histoire,
Geneva*)

really sick. Walked and grew better. Dined at Nyon with French officers. Came to Geneva at five . . . Curious were my thoughts on entering this seat of Calvinism. I put up Aux Trois Rois. I sent immediately to Cazenove, Clavière et Fils for my letters. Young Cazenove brought me a good packet, which made me a very happy man. I had letters from the Margrave of Baden-Durlech, from Rousseau, from Temple, and from Erskine.[1] What a group of ideas! I supped at the *table d'hote*, where was a Monsieur de la Lale, a Parisian, with whom I chatted agreeably.

Sunday, 23 December. I slept till near nine, and sung and was gay even at the seat of Presbyterianism on a Sunday. At two, another young Cazenove came and conducted me to the Eglise de St Germain, as I wished to see a true Geneva kirk. I found a large, dusty building, a precentor with a black wig like Monsieur Dupont, a 'proposant' a-reading the Bible to the Congregation; in short a perfect Puritanical picture. Cazenove would have put me into a good seat, but a fat old woman would not give up her place. She made me smile with her obstinate rudeness. She was just a Scots gracy (devout auld wife). A Monsieur le Cointe preached a good, sensible discourse. After church we walked on the Bastion Bourgeois, an excellent airy place, where the Genevois and Genevoises assemble. We then waited on Monsieur Gaussen, a banker of this city, whose wife is a hearty Aberdeenshire woman, and then we went to a society of young folk where were Cazenove's sisters. It was rather foolish. But I was amused to see card-playing on a Sunday at Geneva, and a minister rampaging amongst them. O John Calvin, where art thou now?

Monday 24th December. After calling on my bankers, Cazenove, Clavière et Fils, from whom I received payment of a bill granted me by Splitgerber and Daum, and on Chappuis et Fils, to whom I was addressed by Messrs Herries and Cochrane, I took a coach for Ferney, the seat of the illustrious Monsieur de Voltaire. I was in true spirits; the earth was covered with snow; I surveyed wild nature with a noble eye. I called up all the grand ideas which I have entertained of Voltaire. The first object that struck me was his church with this inscription: *Deo erexit Voltaire MDCCLXI*. His chateau was handsome. I was received by two or three footmen, who showed me into a very elegant room. I sent by one of them a letter to Monsieur de Voltaire

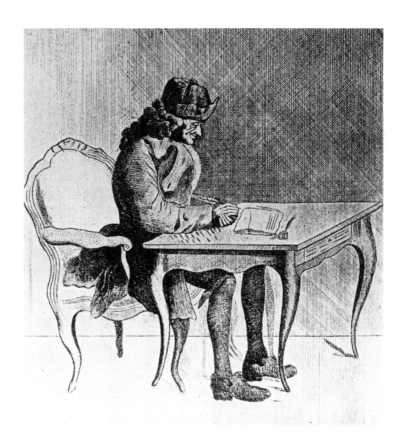

Voltaire at his desk
(from an etching by
Captain Adam)

which I had from Colonel Constant at the Hague. He
returned and told me, 'Monsieur de Voltaire is very much
annoyed at being disturbed. He is abed.' I was afraid that I
should not see him. Some ladies and gentlemen arrived, and
I was entertained for some time. At last Monsieur de Voltaire
opened the door of his apartment, and stepped forth. I
surveyed him with eager attention, and found him just as his
print had made me conceive him. He received me with
dignity, and that air of the world which a Frenchman
acquires in such perfection. He had a slate-blue, fine frieze
greatcoat night-gown,[2] and a three-knotted wig. He sat erect
upon his chair and simpered when he spoke. He was not in
spirits, nor I neither. All I presented was the 'foolish face of
wondering praise'. We talked of Scotland. He said the
Glasgow editions were 'très belles'.[3] I said 'An Academy of

Painting was also established there, but it did not succeed. Our Scotland is no country for that.' He replied with a keen archness, 'No; to paint well it is necessary to have warm feet. It's hard to paint when your feet are cold.' Another would have given a long dissertation on the coldness of our climate. Monsieur de Voltaire gave the very essence of raillery in half a dozen words.

I mentioned the severe criticism which the *Gazette litteraire* has given upon Lord Kames's *Elements*. I imagined it to be done by Voltaire, but would not ask him. He repeated me several of the *bons mots* in it, with an air that confirmed me in my idea of his having written this criticism. He called my Lord always 'ce Monsieur Kames'.

I told him that Mr Johnson and I intended to make a tour through the Hebrides, the Northern Isles of Scotland. He smiled, and cried, 'Very well; but I shall remain here. You will allow me to stay here?' 'Certainly.' 'Well then, go, I have no objections at all.' I asked him if he still spoke English. He replied, 'No. To speak English one must place the tongue between the teeth, and I have lost my teeth.'

He was curious to hear anecdotes from Berlin. He asked who was our Minister there. I said we had only a *chargé d'affaires*. 'Ah!' said he, 'un chargé d'affaires est guère chargé.' He said Hume was 'a true philosopher'.[4]

As we talked, there entered Père Adam, a French Jesuit, who is protected in the house of Voltaire. What a curious idea. He was a lively old man with white hair. Voltaire cried in English, 'There, Sir, is a young man, a scholar who is learning your language, a broken soldier of the Company of Jesus.' 'Ah' said Pere Adam, 'a young man of sixty'.

Monsieur de Voltaire did not dine with us. Madame Denis, his niece, does the honours of his house very well. She understands English. She was remarkably good to me. I sat by her and we talked much. I became lively and most agreeable. We had a company of about twelve. The family consists of seven. The niece of the great Corneille lives here.[5] She is married to Monsieur Dupuits. The gates of Geneva shut at five, so I was obliged to hasten away after dinner without seeing any more of Monsieur de Voltaire.

At Geneva I called for Monsieur Constant Pictet, for whom I had a letter from his sister-in-law, Madame d'Hermenches. I found his lady, who asked me to stay the evening. There was a company here at cards. I saw a

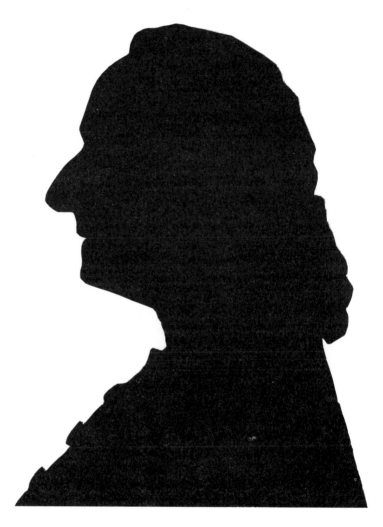

Paper-cut silhouette
presumed to be of Jean-
Jacques Rousseau, *c*.
1765–70 (*Collection
Musée d'art et
d'histoire, Geneva*)

specimen of Genevoises, and compared them with
Rousseau's drawings of them. Constant, the husband, was
lively without wit and polite without being agreeable. There
was a good many men here who railed against Rousseau on
account of his *Lettres écrites de la montagne*. Their fury was
a high farce to my philosophic mind. One of them was arrant
idiot enough to say of the illustrious author 'He's a brute with
brains, a horse with brains, an ox with brains'. 'Rather, a
snake', said a foolish female with a lisping tone. Powers of
absurdity! did your influence ever extend farther? I said 'On

my word, it is time for me to leave this company. Can *women* speak against the author of the *Nouvelle Héloise*?' . . . Madame Constant was an acquaintance of Lord Erskine's. He said he had seen Voltaire morning and evening during a severe sickness, and Mme. Pictet, his wife, had watched him, and he was 'toujours tranquille'. I supped here.

Tuesday, 25 December. Although this was Christmas Day, I fairly fasted, nor stirred out of doors except a moment to the Eglise de St Pierre, which was formerly a Catholic church and is a handsome building. Worship was over, but I heard a voluntary upon the organ. I was in supreme spirits, and a noble idea arose in my mind: I wrote a very lively letter to Madame Denis, begging to be allowed to sleep a night under the roof of Monsieur de Voltaire. I sent it by an express, and Voltaire wrote the answer in the person of his niece, making me very welcome. My felicity this night was abundant. My letter with the answer to it are most carefully preserved.

[Boswell to Madame Denis] *Geneva*, 25 December 1764

I address myself to you, Madam, as to the friend of the stranger. I have the honour of knowing you to be such from most agreeable experience; for yesterday at dinner you not only entertained me with easy and cheerful conversation, but took care that I should have a double portion of the sweet tart which I am so extremely fond of. You may remember, Madam, that I expressed my affection for that dish in the strongest manner: 'Je suis attaché à la tourte'. I spoke in character, for I spoke with that honest frankness with which I declare my sentiments on great and on small occasions. At no time shall I ever envy my faith, my friend, my mistress or my tart.

I present myself in my natural character, which I find suits me the best of any. I own that I have in some periods of my life assumed the characters of others whom I admired. But, as David found the armour of Saul, I found them by much too heavy for me, and, like David, was embarrassed and unable to move with freedom. I hope, Madam, I may be allowed to quote the Old Testament once to the niece of a gentleman who has quoted it so often.

I do not, however, think lightly of my own character. No, Madam, I am proud enough. The French say, 'Proud as a Scotsman'. It shall not be my fault if that proverb goes out of use.

I must beg your interest, Madam, in obtaining for me a

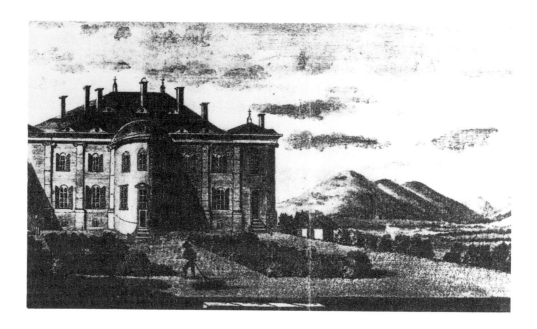

Voltaire's house at Ferney, an anonymous English engraving (from *The Gentleman's magazine, and historical chronicle* of March 1789)

very great favour from Monsieur de Voltaire. I intend to have the honour of returning to Ferney Wednesday or Thursday. The gates of this sober city shut at a most early, I had very near said a most absurd, hour, so that one is obliged to post away after dinner before the illustrious landlord has had time to shine upon his guests. Besides, I believe Monsieur de Voltaire is in opposition to our sun, for he rises in the evening. Yesterday he shot forth some rays. Some bright sparks fell from him. I am happy to have seen so much. But I greatly wish to behold him in full blaze.

Is it then possible, Madam, that I may be allowed to lodge one night under the roof of Monsieur de Voltaire? I am a hardy and a vigorous Scot. You may mount me to the highest and coldest garret. I shall not even refuse to sleep upon two chairs in the bedchamber of your maid. I saw her pass through the room where we sat before dinner.

I beg you let me know if the favour which I ask is granted, that I may bring a nightcap with me. I would not presume to think of having my head honoured with a nightcap of Monsieur de Voltaire. I should imagine that, like the invisible cap of Fortunatus, or that of some other celebrated magician, it would immediately convey to me the qualities of its master; and I own to you, Madam, my head is not strong enough to bear them. His poetical cap I might perhaps support; but his philosophical one would make me so giddy that I should not know which way to turn myself. All I can offer in return for the favour which I ask is many, many thanks; or if Monsieur de Voltaire's delicate French ear would not be offended, I might perhaps offer him a few good rough English verses. Pray, Madam, give me your interest. I would also beg the assistance of my Reverend Father the young man of sixty, the student of our language, the disbanded soldier of the Company of Jesus. Sure a lady and a priest must prevail.

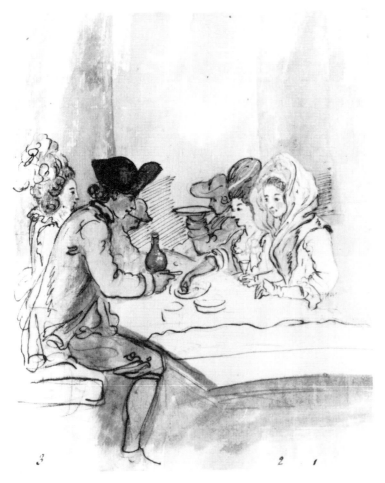

The Meal, by Jean Huber (*Collection Musée d'art et d'histoire, Geneva*)

I have the honour to be, Madam, your very humble servant, Boswell.

As may be guessed, Boswell's night spent under Voltaire's roof was entirely successful – or so we gather from his journal. Boswell at some stage raised the subject with Voltaire of his religious beliefs.

> . . . I talked to him serious and earnest. I demanded of him an honest confession of his real sentiments. He gave it me with candour and with a mild eloquence which touched my heart. I did not believe him capable of thinking in the manner that he declared to me was 'from the bottom of his heart'. He expressed his veneration – his love – for the Supreme Being, and his entire resignation to the will of Him who is All-wise. He expressed his desire to resemble the Author of Goodness by being good himself. His sentiments go no farther. He does not inflame his mind with grand hopes of the immortality of the soul. He says it may be, but he knows nothing of it. And his mind is in perfect tranquility. I was moved; I was sorry. I doubted his sincerity. I called to him with emotion, 'Are you sincere? Are you really sincere?' He answered, 'Before God, I am.' Then with the fire of him whose tragedies have so often shone on the theatre of Paris, he said, 'I suffer much. But I suffer with patience and resignation; not as a Christian but as a man.'
>
> I departed from this chateau in a most extraordinary humour, thinking hard, and wondering if I could possibly, when again in Scotland, again feel my most childish prejudices. When I got to Geneva, I was visited by young Chappuis, to whom I said, 'Monsieur de Voltaire is a poet, he is a sublime poet, and goes very high. Monsieur Rousseau is a philosopher, and goes very deep. One flies, the other plunges.' This is clumsily said, but the thought is not bad. I supped at Monsieur Gaussen's, where I found Lord Stanhope and Lord Abingdon and his brother. I was so-so. I had first been at Professor Maurice's, where I saw his lady, his son, and his daughter.
>
> *Sunday 30 December*. I sat at home all forenoon writing. At three Professor Maurice called upon me and sat an hour. We were cheerful. It was a curious idea: This is a Geneva minister. I talked vastly well, yet I talked of my gloom with pride. He was amazed at it. He asked my correspondence. I

shall write to him. Vanneck[6] was now at Geneva with his
good governor, Monat, who invited me this afternoon to the
société of his wife. He lives in the Maison de Ville. I found
here a very genteel company with true Geneva looks. After
tea and coffee was a ball. The fiddle or fiddles fairly played
and the company fairly danced. Was not this enough to break
my most stubborn association of gloom with a Sunday at
Geneva? To complete the thing, there was a clergyman in
the company. This is the second young Geneva minister that
I have seen. I do not at all like them. I know not if they are
Arians and Socinians, but I am sure they are fops. I played a
hand at whist, and after we had played and danced enough,
we went to supper. I say *we* danced, for although I was not
much in spirits, I danced a minuet with Madame Rilliet,
whom I had seen and grown fond of.

Two years later, the meticulous and (until now) apparently
humourless natural scientist, Thomas Pennant, paid his own visit
to Voltaire. Living up to Dr Johnson's comment on his powers of
observation, he noted:

In the afternoon of the 6th of this month [May] I went with
Mr Martin[7] to visit the celebrated M. de Voltaire at his seat
at Ferney in the Country of Gex . . .
    The first landed property Voltaire had was this place,
where he purchased an extensive manor . . . It commands a
fine view of a flat country well cultivated: Mount Jura, part
of the lake of Geneva and the snowy Alps of Savoy. We were
at first introduced to his niece, Mademoiselle Denis, a
sedate, worthy looking woman about fifty. Voltaire made his
appearance out of an adjacent study, and came into the room
with more affectation of bodily infirmity than was requisite;
not but that he was really as meagre and as arid a figure as
ever I saw. His dress was a sky blue ratteen coat, lapelled, a
blue turned up cap over a long flowing brigadier grey wig,
his knees without buckles, his stocking coarse, his shoes
thick and large. After a short address on the honour we did a
weakly old man, his countenance brightened, his eyes, which
were the most brilliant I ever saw, sparkled with pleasure at
the attention paid to his fame. He repaid with interest our
flattering visit; spoke in our own language, which he seemed
almost to have forgotten except our imprecations, which he
denounced most liberally on himself if he did not love the

English, aye better than his own country-men: By G – I do lov Ingles G – G – dammee, if I don't lov them bettre dan de French G – .' Our victories had made a full impression on the old man. He proposed a walk into his garden, which was extensive but in wretched taste, – with strait walks and espalier hedges, but as it was not inclosed with a wall he informed us that it was flung open in conformity to the English taste. His avarice appeared in his very walks, which were now in mowing for hay, and would have been inaccessible by reason of the grass a few days before. When we returned into the house we found assembled a niece of M. Corneille [i.e. the great-grand-daughter of the uncle of

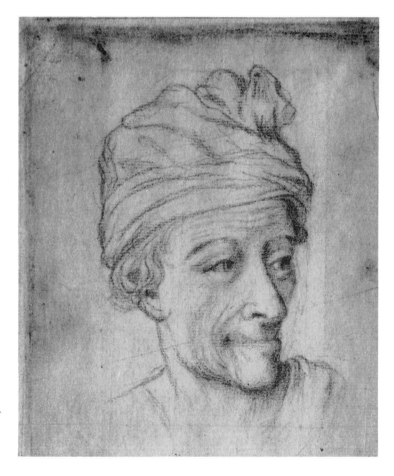

Voltaire, by Jean Huber
(*Cabinet des Dessins,
Collection Musée d'art
et d'histoire, Geneva*)

Corneille], whom he had just married to a pert young Frenchman (Monsieur Dupuits), and portioned with a new edition of her uncle's works; a gentleman from Geneva, the poor skeleton Le Père Adam (a Jesuit whom Voltaire had taken into his household) his constant but, and mademoiselle Denis. A finical young monk joined us. No sooner had the latter entered than Voltaire instantly attacked him, wondering at his imprudence at venturing into the company of the damned; – 'You see, sir, two Englishmen of the reformed church whom you must allow are in a state of damnation: a Genevese Calvinist not a bit better, Le Père Adam, a Jesuit damned at least in France[8], and myself a free thinker. So Reverend sir, let me beg you to retire from such dangerous society.' His conversation was the whole time extremely lively, for fortunately for us this was not one of his gloomy days, when as I was informed he was captious and disagreeable to a high degree. His theatre at this time down; his theatrical entertainments were formerly very frequent. He performed his own pieces and usually acted a part himself. Adjacent to his house is one half of the parish church. He had pulled down the other, and giving the remainder a new front, had the assurance to put in golden letters, – *Deo erexit Voltaire*. The Easter of 1768 was distinguished by the strange Phaenomenon of the appearance of the Lord of the manor at church, where he confessed, received the sacrament, and to the great amazement of the Congregation mounted the pulpit and gave them a sermon on the sin and danger of theft. It seems Voltaire had just been robbed, and hoped by this means to detect the offender. The Clergy were dreadfully scandalized at the profanation. His diocesan, the Archbishop of Anneci, wrote to him three pious and sensible letters, which the wit answered with his usual vivacity. The Prelate finding him incorrigible, applied to the Court, who interfered, took the part of the church and mortified poor Voltaire with obliging him to make and sign the most ample confession of the Catholic faith that was ever penned; to receive the communion and repeat the creed before proper witnesses. He could not forbear even in the action of taking the Viaticum a raillery on the notion of the real presence, declaring with great gravity, 'that having now his God in his mouth he sincerely pardoned all his calumniators', after which the persecution dropped and Voltaire resumed his

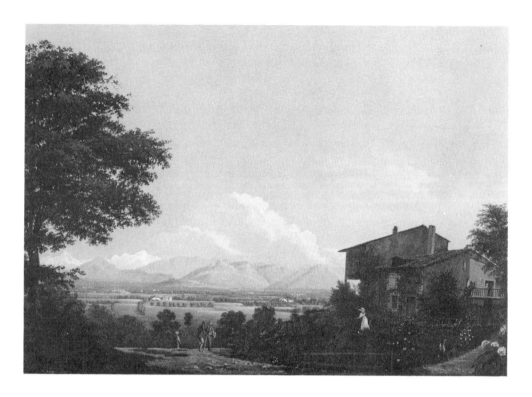

The Mont Blanc range seen from Mornex by Jean DuBois, early nineteenth century (*Collection Musée d'art et d'histoire, Geneva*)

former libertinism, but took especial care never again to appear on the pulpit stage.

Among the constant stream of visitors to Ferney was, of course, John Moore. In the same easy, natural style in which he described Geneva, in *A View of Society and Manners in France, Switzerland and Germany* . . . , he wrote to his patron in 1773, giving a perceptive account of Voltaire and his way of life.

> . . . I am not surprised that your inquiries of late entirely regard the philosopher of Ferney. This extraordinary person has contrived to excite more curiosity, and to retain the attention of Europe for a longer space of time, than any other man this age has produced. Since I have been in this country, I have had frequent opportunities of conversing with him, and still more with those who have lived in intimacy with him for many years; so that, whatever remarks I may send you on this subject, are founded either on my own observation, or on that of the most candid and

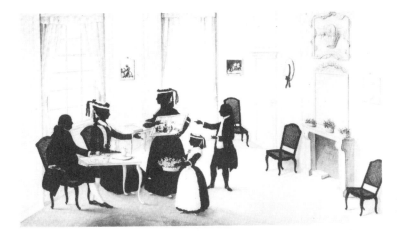

Paper-cut sihouette of Marc Marcet and his family, by Christian-Gottlob Geissler, *c.* 1780 (*Cabinet des Dessins, Collection Musée d'art et d'histoire, Geneva*)

intelligent of his acquaintance . . . The first idea which has presented itself to all who have attempted a description of his person, is that of a skeleton . . . but it must be remembered, that this skeleton, this mere composition of skin and bone, has a look of more spirit and vivacity, than is generally produced by flesh and blood, however blooming and youthful.

The most piercing eyes I ever beheld are those of Voltaire, now in his eightieth year. His whole countenance is expressive of genius, observation, and extreme sensibility.

In the morning he has a look of anxiety and discontent; but this gradually wears off . . . yet an air of irony never entirely forsakes his face . . .

Composition is his principal amusement. No author who writes for daily bread, no young poet ardent for distinction, is more assiduous with his pen, or more anxious for fresh fame, than the wealthy and applauded Seigneur of Ferney.

He lives in a very hospitable manner, and takes care always to keep a good cook. He has generally two or three visitors from Paris, who stay with him a month or six weeks at a time. When they go, their places are soon supplied; so that this is a constant rotation of society at Ferney . . .

All who bring recommendations from his friends, may depend upon being received, if he be not really indisposed.

The forenoon is not a proper time to visit Voltaire. He cannot bear to have his hours of study interrupted. This alone is sufficient to put him in bad humour; besides, he is then apt to be querulous, whether he suffers by the infirmities of age or from some accidental cause of chagrin . . .

Those who are invited to supper, have an opportunity of seeing him in the most advantageous point of view. He then exerts himself to entertain the company, and seems as fond of saying, what are called good things, as ever: – and when any lively remark or *bon mot* comes from another, he is equally delighted, and pays the fullest tribute of applause. – The spirit of mirth gains upon him by indulgence. – When surrounded by his friends, and animated by the preference of women, he seems to enjoy life with all the sensibility of youth . . .

His dislike to the clergy is well known. – This leads him to join in a very trite topic of abuse with people who have no pretention to that degree of wit which alone could make their railings tolerable. The conversation happening to turn into this channel, one person said, If you subtract pride from priests, nothing will remain. – 'Vous comptez donc, Monsieur, la gourmandise pour rien?' ['Then you count greediness for nothing?'] said Voltaire.

In another letter to the Duke of Hamilton, Moore continues:

. . .Voltaire's criticisms on the writings of Shakespeare do him no honour; they betray an ignorance of the author, whose works he so rashly condemns . . . Voltaire's national prejudices, and his imperfect knowledge of the language, render him blind to some of the most shining beauties of the English Poet . . .

Voltaire had formerly a little theatre at his own house . . . Mr Cramer of Geneva sometimes assisted upon these occasions – I have often seen that gentleman act at a private theatre in that city with deserved applause.

The celebrated Clairon herself has been proud to tread Voltaire's domestic theatre, and to display at once his genius and her own . . . I have been frequently at this theatre. The performers are moderately good. The admired Le Kain,[9] who is now at Ferney, on a visit to Voltaire, sometimes exhibits: – but when I go, my chief inducement is to see Voltaire, who generally attends when Le Kain acts, and when one of his own tragedies is to be represented.

He sits on the stage, and behind the scenes; but so as to be seen by a great part of the audience . . . He seems perfectly chagrined and disgusted when any of the actors commit a mistake; and when he thinks they perform well, never fails to mark his approbation with all the violence of voice and gesture.

He enters into the feigned distresses of the piece with every symptom of real emotion, and even sheds tears with the profusion of a girl present for the first time at a tragedy.

One of Voltaire's close companions was the witty and satirical Jean Huber (1723–86). William Beckford, who visited Geneva for the first time at the age of seventeen, found him the best possible company. In a letter to his sister, Mrs Elizabeth Hervey,[10] headed Geneva, 19 January 1778, Beckford tells her:

The way of living at Geneva is far from gay; but in return it is very improving. The Societies are composed of so many clever people that notwithstanding a certain form and solemnity . . . they do not altogether displease me. Another circumstance I like, is the number of original Characters to be met with here. In the first rank of these, shines my Friend Huber whose particular excellence would be very hard to discover, as he is as changeable as the wind and sometimes as boisterous. One day he wanders with his Faucons over Hill and Dale, marsh and river, wood and garden; the next, shut up in his Cabinet he will reflect on the nature of the Universe and the first principle of all things. The following week perhaps he is totally engaged in drawing caricatures and saying the queerest drollest things imaginable . . . See him the day after this whim has left him and you will find a profound Musician, composing *Misereres* and declaiming Recitative with the taste and judgement of an eminent professor . . .

The next Night very likely he would be seen sunk in his Armchair by the Fire side covered with snuff and strewing it about whenever he moves . . . He is now as indolent as you please and seems to have forgot all that activity of Mind and Body for which he is sometimes so remarkable. He will now read nothing but romances and if anybody comes in speaks Spanish. Those who have been with him once before . . . might wish to take up the converation again . . . Let them question him a little – it will be all in vain. He will gape and whistle and pick his teeth and stir the fire. Suppose they persevere. He continues so obstinate that at last quite impatient they ask if he ever heard of the *Etre Suprême*. With all the *sang froid* and gravity conceivable he will answer, *Oui, j'ai entendu dire du bien de lui*.

Farm-buildings outside Geneva, by Huber the Elder (*Cabinet des Dessins, Collection Musée d'art et d'histoire, Geneva*)

And so on. Beckford completes his description:

There are more strange Animals at Geneva besides the one I have attempted to say something about; but there were none so wonderful. You must live with Huber, to be able to

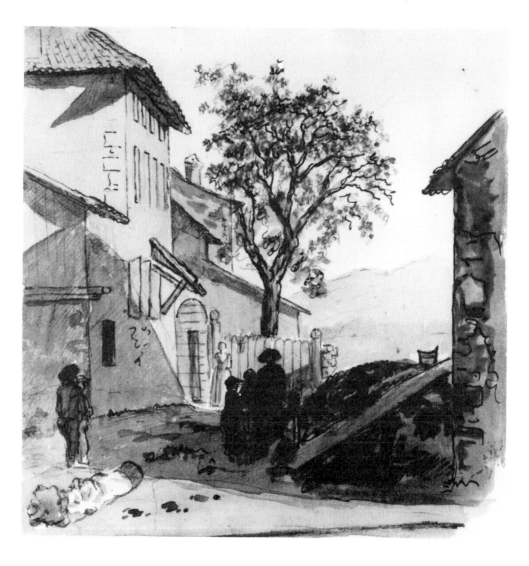

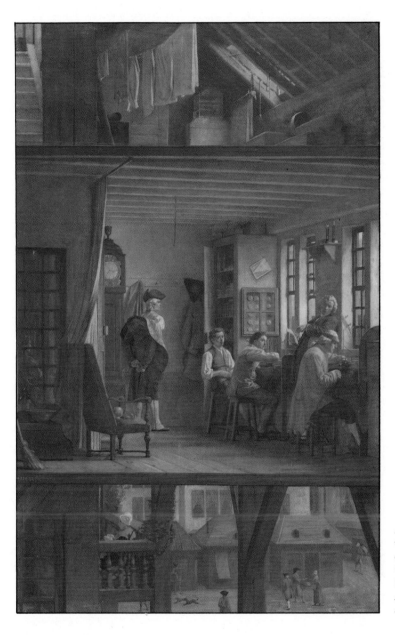

A watchmaker's
workshop in eighteenth-
century Geneva, by
Christophe-François de
Ziegler (*Collection
Musée d'art et
d'histoire, Geneva*)

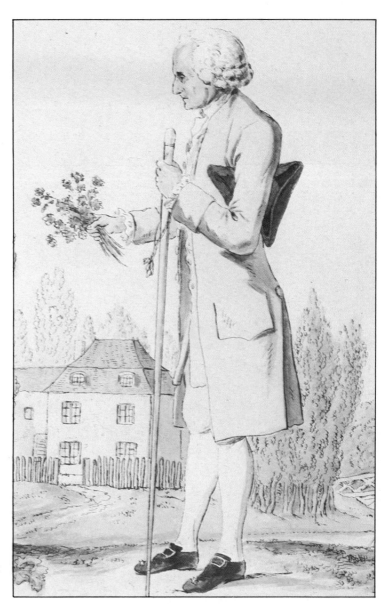

Jean-Jacques Rousseau
botanizing; an
anonymous pen drawing
(*Photograph: Nicolas
Bouvier*)

discern his real perfection, and I greatly fear I have sent you
but a very feeble Sketch. . . .

Jean Huber was born in 1723, the son of a member of the
Genevese Council of 200. His uncle was the Abbé Huber, whose
Mémoires intrigued Voltaire (alas, they have long ago disappeared), and his aunt was a theologian and philanthropist of
note. As a young man Huber spent some time as an ensign in the
grenadiers at the Court of the Landgrave Charles de Hesse-
Cassel, and later at that of Charles-Emmanuel, king of Sardinia.
From early on he had shown himself to be a skilled artist and
this, together with his interest in falconry and an unusual wit,
made him predictably popular with princes.

In 1746, he returned to Geneva and married Marie-Louise
Alleon, cousin to Madame Necker, mother of Madame de Staël.
Barely thirty, he was soon elected to the Council of 200. Shortly
after the birth of Huber's second son, in October 1754, Voltaire
decided to settle in Geneva. At first, this distinguished personality, known to be somewhat disenchanted with Catholicism,
was received with open arms. From the beginning, he entertained
lavishly; the Genevese, and a host of foreign visitors, poured into
his property at Ferney. However, he depended on witty com-
panionship and when Councillor Tronchin introduced Huber to
him, he quickly began to find him indispensable. From then
onwards, Huber was always fetched when anyone of real importance arrived. On these occasions, he fell into the habit of making
a host of small, satirical sketches of Voltaire – sketches which
encompassed the philosopher's every mood and which frequently
included the crowned heads and aristocracy of Europe. It was in
1760 that Voltaire moved to Ferney, and in this same year Huber
discovered the art of the *découpure* (paper-cut silhouette).

This new form of art had become the rage in Paris and
thereafter spread rapidly through Europe. However, nobody
could equal Huber in brilliance of execution and Grimm, who
happened to be in Geneva, became fascinated by his achieve-
ments, thereafter singing his praises everywhere. Catherine the
Great, the English Court, Gustaf III of Sweden, the Duchess of
Saxe-Weimar, the Marquise du Deffand, to whom Voltaire
complained that Huber was ridiculing him: all were enchanted
with Huber's *découpure*, centred as it was almost entirely on the
idiosyncrasies of Voltaire. (Madame du Deffand, in fact, sent
examples to Horace Walpole.)

Having recorded views of the 'Sage of Ferney' (many of them, amazingly, cut out with scissors and paper held either behind his back or under the table), at all hours of the day and night, over a period of ten years, Huber turned his hand to painting him. Most of these resulting works went to Catherine the Great, who had told him she would accept anything he did, and the more there were, the better.

In May 1772, Huber left with his family for Paris. Voltaire, finding himself suddenly without 'his' artist and missing his company, gave vent to his irritation in petulant letters to friends. The reason for this Parisian journey was a tragic one. Huber's eldest son, François, was losing his sight and his father hoped to find a cure for him in the French capital. The visit was a failure and François returned to Geneva completely blind, at the age of twenty-two. He was already studying natural history and notably the life of bees. With the aid of his servant Burnens, he was able to continue his research – ultimately becoming known in the international scientific world as 'Huber des Abeilles'. A certain Mademoiselle Lullin, who had loved him since the age of sixteen, approached his father on their return from Paris and asked permission to marry him. This must have much comforted Jean Huber.[11]

On his return from France, nearly a year later, Huber settled down for most of the time in a house in Cologny with magnificent views to the north and south. He continued to make sketches and paintings of Voltaire, but these were for the most part from memory. From now on he went less and less to Geneva, for by now many of his friends had moved to Paris. There was no quarrel between him and Voltaire; the distance between Cologny and Ferney could be regarded as largely responsible for this apparent 'cooling off'.

Voltaire died in 1778, and Jean Huber, who had probably known him most intimately, almost certainly missed him more than anyone.[12]

Notes

1. William Johnson Temple and the Hon. Andrew Erskine, intimate friends of Boswell's youth.
2. Boswell means that his night-gown (we would say dressing-gown) was cut like a great-coat.
3. Editions of the classics published in Glasgow by Robert Andrew Foulis.
4. David Hume. Scottish philosopher with whose sceptical views

on religion Boswell thoroughly disagreed. It was he who invited Rousseau to London in 1766.

5. 'The niece of the great Corneille', described more accurately by Pennant's editor, in the account of his visit two years later as 'the great-grand-daughter of the uncle of Corneille'.

6. Sir Joshua Vanneck. A prominent London merchant.

7. Mr Martin is described by Valltravers as 'of Worcestershire, at the Temple'.

8. Jesuits had been proscribed in France since 1762.

9. Le Kain. Celebrated actor.

10. *The Life and Letters of William Beckford*, Lewis Melville: Heinemann, 1910.

11. This incident was recounted by Voltaire in a letter to Madame Necker. He finishes typically: 'Ce serait Psyche amoureuse de l'Amour, si ces deux enfants etaient plus jolis!' [It would be Psyche in love with Love, if these two children were better-looking!']

12. Summary and translation of extracts from G. Jean-Aubury's article, *Jean Huber ou le Démon de Genève*, in the *Revue de Paris*, May-June 1936.

CHAPTER 3

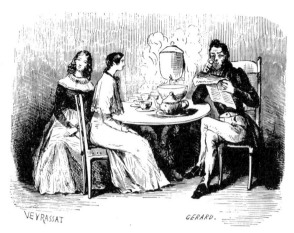

MARIA EDGEWORTH AND THE
BIBLIOTHÈQUE BRITANNIQUE

Seventeen years after Voltaire's death in 1778, the Genevese professor Marc-Auguste Pictet, together with his brother Charles Pictet-de-Rochemont and Frédéric-Guillaume Maurice, founded a new scientific and literary periodical in Geneva, the *Bibliothèque Britannique*, which in 1816 changed its name to the *Bibliothèque Universelle*.[1] The motives behind its launching were varied; it has even been suggested that amongst them was a desire on the part of the editors to irritate the French by their choice of title and content. In 1795, the date of the first issue of the *Bibliothèque Britannique*, it noted the arrival on the literary scene of Maria Edgeworth, (1767–1849) the Anglo-Irish moralistic writer: and in 1798 and 1799 it published *Practical Education*, a joint work by Maria and her father, R.L. Edgeworth. This was translated into French by Charles Pictet-de-Rochemont and was highly acclaimed. Thereafter, the *Biblothèque Britannique* published and reviewed everything of Maria's that it could acquire.

Maria Edgeworth's family life and upbringing – principally at Edgeworthstown in Ireland – were at all times distinguished by warmth of affection, intelligence and balanced thought. Her father believed in 'experimental' education:

> . . . The art of teaching to invent – I dare not say, but of awakening and assisting the inventive power by daily exercise and excitement, and by the application of

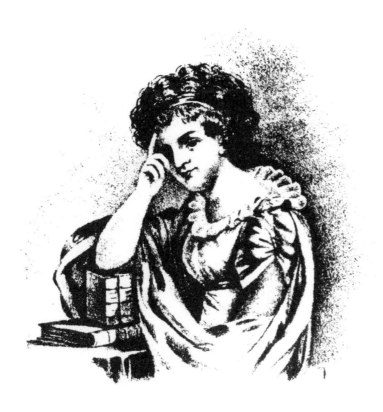

Engraving of Maria
Edgeworth, frontispiece
to Augustus Hare's *The
Life and Letters of
Maria Edgeworth*, 1894

philosophic principles to trivial occurrences – he [my father]
believed might be pursued with infinite advantage to the
rising generation.

Maria was the second in a large family, her own mother and first
step-mother dying young. Maria had a vivid imagination and a
capacity for letter-writing demonstrated in the splendid collection
of her letters to her much-loved family. Her father encouraged her
literary tendencies from an early age. In 1795 she published *Letters
for Literary Ladies* and this was followed in 1796 by *The Parents*.
Mrs Elizabeth Edgeworth, Maria's second stepmother, died
tragically in 1797, after seventeen years of being the family pivot –
thus leaving her husband with a large family, all of whom were
living at home. The following year Mr Edgeworth, clearly not
destined for widowerhood, married for the fourth time. He seems
to have been an excellent chooser of stepmothers, as once again

his children were wisely and devotedly cared for. As for Maria, she and her new stepmother soon became close friends. The marriage was within days of the Irish rebellion which preceded the French invasion; and in a letter a few days afterwards to her favourite aunt, Mrs Ruxton, Maria describes the family flight from Edgeworthstown in the path of the French, and of their enforced stay at an inn at Longford.

Later that year, Maria and her father published their first joint work – *Practical Education. Castle Rackrent*, Maria's first novel, was published two years later, followed soon after by *Belinda*, and it was at about this time that Edgeworthstown received a visit from the Genevese professor, Marc-Auguste Pictet.

Pictet paid visits to England and Ireland in the summer of 1801 and published an account of his travels in the *Bibliothèque Britannique* the following year. He gives this description of Maria:

I had persuaded myself that the author of the work on Education, and of other productions, useful as well as ornamental, would betray herself by a remarkable exterior. I was mistaken. A small figure, eyes nearly always lowered, a profoundly modest and reserved air, with expression in the features when not speaking: such was the result of my first survey. But when she spoke, which was too rarely for my taste, nothing could have been better thought, and nothing better said, though always timidly expressed, than that which fell from her mouth.

In fact, Mr Edgeworth allowed Pictet small opportunity to converse with Maria. According to H.W. Hausermann in *The Genevese Background*, Pictet wrote in the *Bibliothèque Britannique* that Maria's father had monopolised his attention. 'Que imagineroit-on que fut le premier sujet de conversation lancé par Mr E.? "Jusqu'a quel degré présumez-vous," me dit-il, "qu'un gazomètre puisse déterminer la préssion exercée sur un fluide élastique?" . . . Il se termina heureusement avec le dejeuner.' ('What would you imagine was the first subject of conversation raised by Mr E.? "To what degree," he said to me, "can a gasometer calculate the pressure exercised on an elastic fluid?" . . . Luckily, he finished with the arrival of lunch.') When at long last Pictet was free to discuss '*divers sujets de morale*' with Maria, it appears that he did most of the talking.

Unfortunately Pictet was only able to spend one day in

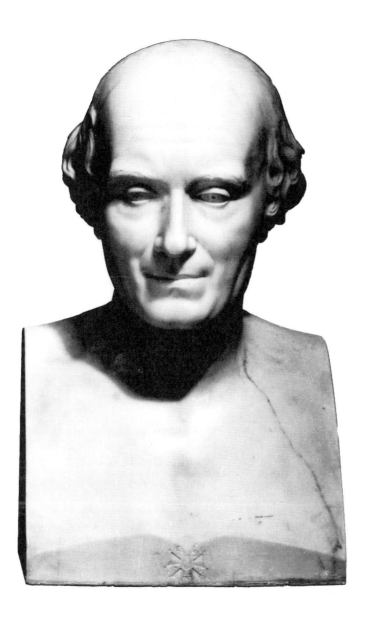

Bust of Marc-Auguste
Pictet by James Pradier
(*MAH, Geneva;
Collection Societé des
Arts*)

Edgeworthstown. Before leaving, however, he persuaded Mr Edgeworth to make a visit to Geneva, spending some time in Paris on the way. In the event, the Edgeworths arrived on the Continent at the end of October 1802, to find that, *grâce aux Pictets* and the *Bibliothèque Britannique*, they were the centre of attraction in literary circles. In Paris, the Delessert family[2] introduced them into intellectual and fashionable society, and before long they were the focal point of attention and evident appreciation.

In a letter to Mrs Ruxton dated 1 December 1802, Maria writes of Madame Delessert, to whom Pictet had particularly introduced them:

> . . . At Madame Delessert's house there are, and have been for years, meetings of the most agreeable and select society in Paris: she has the courage absolutely to refuse to admit either man or woman whose conduct she cannot approve; at other houses there is sometimes a strange mixture. To recommend Madame Delessert still more powerfully to you, I must tell you that she was the benefactress of Rousseau; he was, it is said, never good or happy except in her society: To her bounty he owed his retreat in Switzerland.

Later, writing to her aunt, Mrs Mary Sneyd about Madame Houdetot, (who had evidently inspired Rousseau to create 'Julie'):

> . . . I wish I could at seventy-two be such a woman! She told me that Rousseau, while he was writing so finely on education, and leaving his own children in the Foundling Hospital, defended himself with so much eloquence that even those who blamed him in their hearts, could not find tongues to answer him. Once at dinner . . . there was a fine pyramid of fruit. Rousseau in helping himself took the peach which formed the base of the pyramid, and the rest fell immediately. 'Rousseau,' said she, 'that is what you are always doing with all our systems. You pull down with a single touch; but who will build up what you pull down?'[3]

To crown her unquestioned success in Paris, Maria received a proposal of marriage from Monsieur Edelcrantz, the Swedish envoy. Although she stated quite clearly that 'nothing could tempt me to leave my own dear friends and my own country to live in Sweden,' her stepmother felt otherwise.

. . .Maria was mistaken as to her own feelings. She refused
Monsieur Edelcrantz, but she felt much more for him than
esteem and admiration; she was exceedingly in love with him
. . . She decided rightly for her own future happiness and for
that of her family, but she suffered much at the time and
long afterwards.[4]

Maria Edgeworth unquestionably owed her Continental
reputation as a writer to the Pictet brothers and the support they
gave her in their *Bibliothèque Britannique*. At the same time,
while largely applauding her moralistic views on childrens'
education, the Pictets and their readers by no means always
approved of her views. For example, they disliked private
education and disagreed strongly with Maria's doctrine that
children should not come in contact with house-servants. They
also at times found too much worldliness in her philosophy.
Marc-Auguste, however, gave strongest proof of his admiration
and friendship for the Edgeworths by ensuring the warmth of
their welcome in Parisian intellectual circles.

As yet, England was not at war with France, but the following
extract from the London *Times* of 10 April 1798 gives some idea
of the situation of Geneva in relation to France at that period:

. . . *HELVETIA* . . . Switzerland is completely reduced to
subjection; and a REPUBLIC *one and indivisible* has been
substituted, under the irresistible auspices of a French army,
in the place of the ancient Helvetic Confederacy. The new
Administrators of this revolutionary system will no doubt be
appointed in the same *free and unbiased* manner, under the
protection and influence of the Directorial artillery. Thus a
country, which has, for upwards of 200 years, enjoyed an
equal portion of happiness with the freest and most tranquil
part of Europe, is at length given up to all the disorders of
anarchy, and forced to crouch to the falling yoke of a
despotic government. The small Republic, of Geneva, which
entertained some hope of being united with Switzerland,
finding itself placed under the absolute control of France,
has at length been to the necessity of incorporating itself with
the Great Nation.

As Genevese delegate to the Tribunate from 1802 to 1807,
Pictet completely identified himself with the cause of the French
Empire in which the republic of Geneva had been absorbed. In

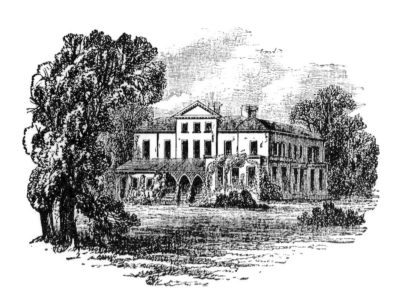

Edgeworthstown (from
*A Study of Maria
Edgeworth* by Grace A.
Oliver, 1882)

1807 he was appointed *Inspecteur général des études de l'empire
français* and, in the following year, *Inspecteur général de
l'université*.[5]

When Napoleon came to Geneva and dined at the home of the
French Resident-General, Marc-Auguste Pictet was placed on his
right. Hausermann points out, however, that his 'activity as a
Frenchman did not prevent his election to the *Conseil
Representatif* of Geneva during the first two years after the city
had regained its freedom and became a canton of the Swiss
Confederation in 1814.'[6]

The outbreak of war between France and England brought the
Edgeworths' stay on the Continent to a precipitate end. They left
Paris at the beginning of 1803, going first to London and then to
Edinburgh, before returning to Ireland. Maria was not to visit
Geneva for another seventeen years.

Back again at Edgeworthstown, Mrs Edgeworth tells us that
Maria threw herself into the preparation of a series of books, and
from then on her letters appear full of lively happenings within
the family, interspersed with news of friends and prominent
personalities.

Tales of Fashionable Life, published in June 1809, was well
received by the public. Once again, however, her moralising tone
is irritating; and indeed it was this publication that led to Madame

de Staël's withering comment to Etienne Dumont: '*Vraiment Miss Edgeworth est digne de l'enthousiasme, mais elle se perd dans votre triste utilite.*' (Miss Edgeworth is really worthy of enthusiasm, but she loses herself in dreary practicality.') Not surprisingly, Maria, who heard of it, could not forgive her.

A second series of *Tales of Fashionable Life* appeared in 1812. Of these 'The Absentee' was a masterpiece and contains one scene which Macaulay declared to be the best thing written of its kind since the opening of the twenty-second book of the *Odyssey*. (Yet Mrs Edgeworth writes that the greater part of 'The Absentee' was 'written under the torture of toothache.'[7])

In 1813, Maria's father and stepmother decided to take her to London for the season. In the event, she was lionised from the first moment, and no sooner had they arrived than the Genevese jurist and writer Etienne Dumont, who happened to be in London, came to see her. She had first met him at the beginning of her original stay in Paris, in 1802. Madame Gautier, daughter of Madame Delessert, had invited the Edgeworths to her country house in Passy. Here they had met, in addition to the Delessert family,

. . . Madame de Pastoret, a literary and fashionable lady . . .

Monsieur de Pastoret, her husband, a man of diplomatic knowledge; Lord Henry Petty, son of Lord Lansdowne, with whom my father had much conversation; the Swiss Ambassador, whose name I will not attempt to spell; Monsieur Dumont,[8] a Swiss gentleman, travelling with Lord Henry Petty, very sensible and entertaining, I am sorry that he has since left Paris . . .

Now, in London, Maria gives an unflattering physical portrait of him in a letter to her cousin Sophie Ruxton.

. . . A fattish, Swiss-looking man in black with monstrous eyebrows and a large red face like what the little robbins described the gardener's face when it looked down upon them in their nest – I felt at once *que l'amour n'avoit jamais passé et ne passeroit jamais par là.* [I felt at once that love had never and would never be found there.] *Au reste* he is and will be always to us an excellent friend, a man of first-rate abilities, superior in conversation to anyone I have met with except Sir James McIntosh. Dumont leads the life of a French *savant* in society . . . wants nothing more and seems to have sold himself to Bentham as Dr Faustus sold himself to the devil . . .[9]

The family of Humphry Davy in particular overwhelmed the Edgeworths with hospitality in the summer of 1813. Sir Humphry, distinguished chemist and philosopher and inventor of the Davy lamp, had several times met Maria and her family in previous years. He had recently succeeded in marrying a widow to whom he had been laying siege – the rich, sparkling Mrs Apreece. Lady Davy was in full flood that May, giving parties for Maria and introducing her everywhere. It appears that people stood on chairs at assemblies in order to catch a glimpse of her tiny figure. Her stepmother wrote of 'Maria's prominent position . . . visited and noticed as she is by everyone . . .'

When Madame de Staël who was also expected in London at that moment failed to arrive, someone at a large dinner-party asked when she was likely to come. 'Not till Miss Edgeworth is gone,' replied Samuel R . . . 'Madame de Staël would not like two stars shining at the same time.' Immediately a gentleman rose at the end of the table – her son Auguste de Staël. 'Madame de Staël is incapable of such a base thing,' he announced solemnly, before resuming his place.[10]

In 1817 Maria's father died, leaving her the difficult task of completing his *Memoirs*. Maria was devastated, as were all her family, by Richard Edgeworth's death. For some time afterwards, her eyes gave her a great deal of pain and she was scarcely able to read or write. In due course, she managed to finish her father's manuscript and sent it for comments to Etienne Dumont. He had returned to Geneva after the restoration of its independence in 1814 and from there made annual visits to England.

In September 1818, Maria and her sister Honora arrived at Bowood, home of Lord and Lady Lansdowne. Dumont was already a guest there and Maria writes soon after to her stepmother: '. . . Dumont . . . has been very much pleased with my father's MS; he has read a good deal of mine and likes it.' She then gives a description of their days' routine:

After walk, dress and make haste for dinner. Dinner always pleasant, because Lord and Lady Lansdowne converse so agreeably – Dumont also – towards the dessert . . . Dumont read out one evening one of Corneille's plays, *Le Florentin*, beautiful; and beautifully read. We asked for one of Molière, but he said to Lord Lansdowne that it was impossible to read

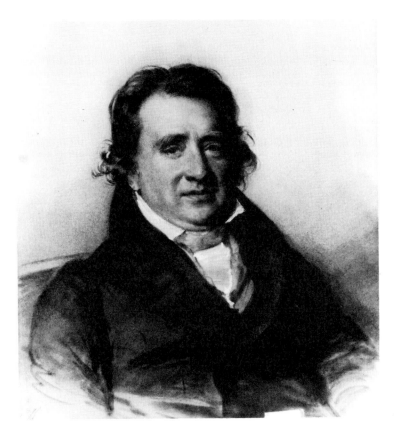

Etienne Dumont, by
Amélie Munier-Romilly
(*Collection Musée d'art
et d'histoire, Geneva*)

out Molière without a quicker eye than he had *pour de
certains propos* [for certain situations]; they went to the
library and brought out at last . . . *Le vieux Célibataire*, an
excellent play . . . and the old bachelor himself a charming
character. Dumont read it as well as Tessier could have read
it, but there were things which seemed as if they were
written on purpose for the Célibataire who was listening, and
the Célibataire who was reading.[11]

In May 1820, Maria returned to Paris for three months,
together with two of her sisters, Fanny and Harriet. Once again
they were received with warmth and admiration in the salons.
Maria's description of Benjamin Constant is ruthless:

. . . I do not like him at all: his countenance, voice, manner

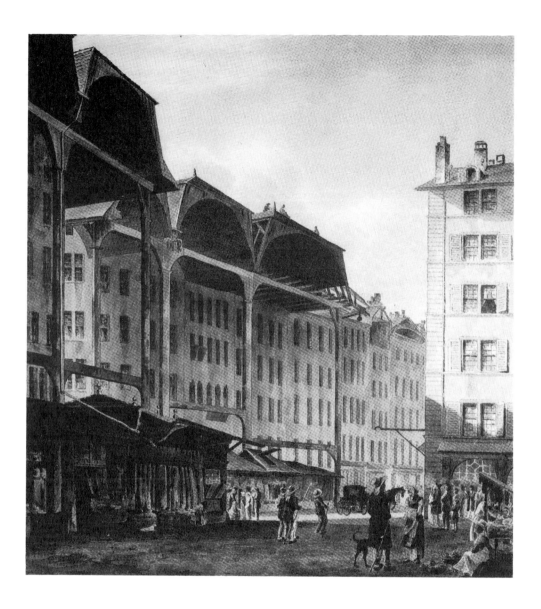

The old rue des Allemands, seen from the place de la Fusterie, artist unknown, 1826–9 (Collection Musée d'art et d'histoire, Geneva)

and conversation are all disagreeable to me. He is a fair, *whithky*-looking man, very near-sighted, with spectacles which seem to pinch his nose. He pokes out his chin to keep the spectacles on, and yet looks over the top of the spectacles, *squinching* up his eyes so that you cannot see your way into his mind . . . He does not give me any confidence in the sincerity of his patriotism, nor any high idea of his talents, though he seems to have a mighty high idea of them himself.[12]

Maria, Fanny and Harriet arrived in Geneva at the beginning of August 1820, staying with her friends the Moillets at Pregny.[13] From then on she saw Dumont constantly, in company with Marc-Auguste Pictet, Dr and Mrs Marcet,[14] and others. Maria was taken on a very successful excursion to Chamonix and on 6 August she writes (to her aunt, Mrs Ruxton):

. . . The day after our return we dined at Mrs. Marcet's with Monsieur Dumont, Monsieur and Madame Prévost, Monsieur de la Rive, Monsieur de Bonstetten, and Monsieur de Candolle, the botanist, a particularly agreeable man. He told us of many experiments on the cure of goitres. In proportion as the land has been cultivated in some districts the goitres have disappeared.

From Pregny, on 10 August 1820, she writes to Mrs Edgeworth:

. . . Dumont, tell Honora, is very kind and cordial; he seems to enjoy universal consideration here, and he loves Mont Blanc next to Bentham, above all created things: I had no idea till I saw him how much he enjoyed the beauties of nature . . .
Dumont speaks to me in the kindest, most tender, and affectionate manner of our *Memoirs*; he says he hears from England, and from all who have read them, that they have produced the effect we wished and hoped; the Ms. had interested him, he said, so deeply that with all his efforts he could not then put himself in the place of the indifferent public . . .
But I must tell you of our visit to Monsieur and Madame de Candolle: we went there to see some volumes of drawings of flowers which had been made for him.

Maria then goes on to relate the story of the remarkable drawings commissioned and paid for in the first instance by Joseph Bonaparte. The Spanish artist/botanist responsible for the drawings found himself without his patron when Joseph was dethroned. He settled in Marseilles, where he met Monsieur de

Candolle. De Candolle, greatly impressed with his work, was able to make constructive suggestions for its improvement. They worked together on it for eighteen months and, when de Candolle was to return to Geneva, the Spaniard said, 'Take the book – as far as I am concerned, I give it to you, but if my government should reclaim it, you will let me have it.' De Candolle took it and returned to Geneva. The following summer he gave a most successful series of lectures on botany. As the course was finishing, he heard from the Spaniard that the King was reinstating him in his previous professorship. He dared not meet the King without his book and therefore asked de Candolle to return it within eight days. One of de Candolle's young lady-pupils was present when he received the letter and expressed his regret at losing the drawings; she exclaimed, 'We will copy them for you.' De Candolle said that it was impossible – 1,500 drawings in eight days! He had some duplicates, however, and some that were not peculiar to Mexico he threw aside; this reduced the number to a thousand, which were distributed among the volunteer artists. The talent and the industry shown, he reported, were astonishing; all joined in this benevolent undertaking without vanity and without rivalship. 'We saw thirteen folio volumes of these drawings done in the eight days!'

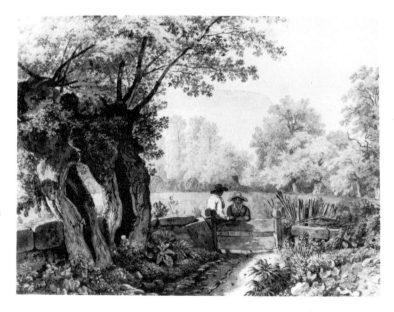

Two peasants talking in the countryside, with the Salève in the background, by A. W. Töpffer (*MAH, Geneva; Collection Societé des Arts*)

Maria, with Fanny and Harriet, then went off on two brief tours of Switzerland with her friends, accompanied by the devoted and competent Monsieur Dumont. Much has been written about their 'Amour d'Automne', though on the whole Maria's biographers and members of the Edgeworth family believe the friendship to have been intellectual and wholly platonic. The frequent and by no means disinterested mention of Dumont's name in Maria's lengthy correspondence with Madame Marcet would appear to belie this. However, the true situation can only be a matter of supposition, and it is important to remember that when Maria met Dumont again in 1820 she had lost her father (with whom she had had a quite exceptional relationship of love and admiration) only three years before. It seems clear that in Dumont she felt she had found another father-figure, with whom she could exchange critical appreciation of books, and who would at all times be comfortingly supportive. In fact, he helped her to prepare her father's *Memoirs* for publication, and she endeavoured to repay him by sending him a detailed *critique* of his book on Bentham, which appeared in 1823.

For many years after the Geneva visit Maria did her best to persuade Dumont to come to Edgeworthstown. Unaware that his health was failing and knowing that he was to be in London in June 1828, she made plans for him to be subsequently conveyed to Edgeworthstown. But Dumont was a sick man and had to return hurriedly to Geneva. When Madame Marcet wrote to break the news of his death, Maria was overwhelmed with grief:

. . . Oct. 25th 1829. Oh my dear Madame Marcet, so many thoughts of mine, so many feelings connected with literature, with my father, with my happiest days! You will allow me kind as you are thus selfishly to speak of my own private loss in the midst even of what as you truly say is a public calamity. I am glad that his own Geneva is so highly sensible of her obligations to him and of his superior merit both of head and heart.

Maria lived until 1849. The flow of letters continued, to her family and to her many close friends – descriptions of her stay with Sir Walter Scott, and of his at Edgeworthstown; visits to the Lansdownes; meetings with Mrs Fry, Sir Humphry Davy, Lady Byron, Mrs Siddons, Darwin. She died aged eighty-two, and in a letter written a few weeks beforehand, wrote:

Our pleasures in literature do not, I think, decline with age; last 1st of January was my eighty-second birthday, and I think that I had as much enjoyment from books as I ever had in my life.

Maria Edgeworth's life was clearly profoundly affected by her Genevan connections. This extraordinary woman was a very model of warm affection and loving concern for her family and close friends; while between her father and herself there existed an intellectual affinity and understanding which seems almost unique. She really was the soul of good nature, sharing in her letters to aunts, stepmother, sisters and cousins all such little details as she knew would give them pleasure. She also appears to have had little conceit where her own gifts are concerned. Yet, she was unquestionably a snob and not only an intellectual one. Writing from Paris to her cousin Sophie Ruxton in 1802, Maria remarks:

> . . . My aunt asks me what I think of French society? All I have seen of it I like extremely, but we hear on all sides that we see only the best of Paris – the men of literature and the *ancienne noblesse. Les nouveaux riches* are quite a different set . . .

On the subject of other literary lights of her generation, she shows herself at times insensitive, intolerant, and even (quite unconsciously) jealous. She thought nothing of Stendhal, for example, and took particular pleasure in Madame Marcet's observation in connection with one of Jane Austen's novels: 'one grows tired at last of milk and water even though the water be pure and the milk sweet.' Byron was anathema to her, as shown in a letter written from Edgeworthstown in April 1810, to C. Sneyd Edgeworth in London:

> I do not like Lord Byron's *English Bards and Scotch Reviewers*, though, as my father says, the lines are very strong, and worthy of Pope and *The Dunciad*. But I was so much prejudiced against the whole by the first lines I opened upon about the 'paralytic muse' of the man who had been his guardian, and is his relation, and to whom he had dedicated his first poems, that I could not relish his wit. He may have great talents, but I am sure he has neither a great nor good mind; and I feel dislike and disgust for His Lordship.

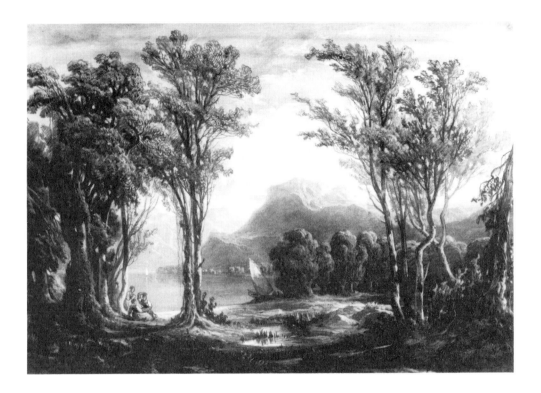

Above all, she both admired and despised Madame de Staël and, as we have seen, could not forgive her for that acid comment on *Tales of Fashionable Life*. By some strange chance, the two women never met, and after Madame de Staël's death in 1817, Maria considerably altered her view of her, influenced at last, perhaps, by Dumont, who had always admired her. When she visited Switzerland in 1820 with her young sisters Fanny and Harriet, they spent what was clearly an agreeable and *sympathique* morning at Coppet with Auguste de Staël and his mother's devoted friend Miss Randall. What undoubtedly pleased her most was that 'Monsieur de Staël and Miss Randall spoke in the most gratifying terms of praise of my father's life.'

View of Lake Geneva by François Diday (*MAH, Geneva; Collection Societé des Arts*)

Notes

1. This publication was to continue, in more or less the same form, until 1924.
2. Benjamin Delessert was a well-known banker and prominent

botanist. A founder-member, with de Candolle, of La Société
Philanthropique.

3. *Life and Letters of Maria Edgeworth*, Volume II, Augustus
    Hare, 1894.
4. *Memoir of Maria Edgeworth* by the late Mrs Edgeworth, edited
    by her children: not published.
5. *The Genevese Background*, H.W. Hausermann, Routledge and
    Kegan Paul Ltd, 1952.
6. Ibid.
7. *Memoir of Maria Edgeworth* by the late Mrs Edgeworth, edited
    by her children.
8. Monsieur Dumont was then tutor to Lord Henry Petty (later
    Marquis of Lansdowne). He translated Bentham's *Traité sur la
    Legislation* and *Théories des Peines et des Récompenses*.
9. Maria Edgeworth detested Bentham's works, which she believed
    were only made understandable by Dumont.
10. *A Study of Maria Edgeworth*, Grace H. Oliver, A. Williams &
    Co., Boston, 1882. The quotation is attributed to Tom Moore.
11. *Memoir of Maria Edgeworth* by the late Mrs Edgeworth, edited
    by her children.
12. *Life and Letters of Maria Edgeworth*, Volume II, Augustus
    Hare, 1894.
13. Madame Moillet was the daughter of Mr Keir, Mrs Edgeworth's
    old friend. They had recently acquired a house on the Lake.
14. Madame Jane Marcet (née Haldimand), 1769–1858, also wrote
    educational books for children. She and Maria Edgeworth
    corresponded regularly for many years (in particular between
    1813 and 1820). Unfortunately only Maria's letters survive.

CHAPTER 4

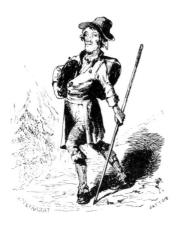

AUGUSTIN-PYRAMUS DE CANDOLLE
AND THE ENGLISH SYSTEMATISTS

Augustin-Pyramus de Candolle, mentioned by Maria Edgeworth on her visit to Geneva in 1820 as 'Monsieur de Candolle . . . a particularly agreeable man', was born on 4 February 1778 (the year of Linnaeus' death). His family had originally come to Geneva from Provence as religious refugees in the sixteenth century and had been Genevese for two hundred years. When de Candolle was eighteen, he went to Paris, having studied briefly there eighteen months earlier. Before he left Geneva, he was much influenced by Monsieur Senébier, who encouraged him to concentrate his studies on vegetal physiology. He tells us revealingly in his *Mémoires* that, together with his close friends, Maurice, Picot and Pictet, he 'formed a small research society, known as the Society of Physical Sciences. This helped to preserve in me some taste for study in the midst of social distractions into which I threw myself with a sort of passion.' Meanwhile, he saw clearly that the freedom of Geneva was doomed, and that it was only a matter of time before it became totally absorbed into the French Republic. It was this, in fact, which eventually decided him to study medicine in Paris.

Although so young, de Candolle was soon accepted as an equal by French scientists of the time. Together with Benjamin Delessert, he was a founder-member of La Société Philanthropique; and he seems to have shone socially, being a regular member of Madame de Rumford's '*brilliant et écléctique*' salon. In spite of his successes, however, he remained devoted to

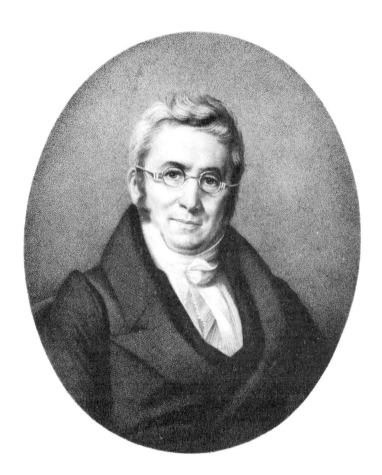

Augustin-Pyramus de
Candolle, by Amélie
Munier-Romilly
(*Bibliothèque Publique
et Universitaire,
Geneva*)

his birthplace, unable to forget how, as an adolescent, he had seen
with anguish Geneva's annexation by France. He had not been
long in Paris when Napoleon gave orders that the *prefets* should
send him, for each department of France, three men who could
explain to him the wishes of their populations. De Candolle was
chosen to be one of the three representing the department of
Léman. 'Well,' asked Bonaparte, 'is Geneva pleased at being
united with France?' 'No, General,' replied de Candolle, 'but
since the 18 *brumaire* she is a little less unhappy.' Napoleon
began, with a certain good humour, to enumerate the advantages
Geneva acquired from the new situation. But he soon saw that his
young listener was not convinced, and made no attempt to appear
so. De Candolle was and remained among the small number of
intellectuals who never benefitted from imperial favours.[1]

During his ten years in Paris, de Candolle spent a large part of his time at the Jardin des Plantes, where he was known as the young man with the watering-can. Botany at this stage was not sufficient for him. He studied enough zoology to be able to give lessons in it later on, and passed his diploma as a doctor. His thesis appropriately was 'The Medical Properties of Plants'. The day he graduated, his – already distinguished – scientist friends, Biot, Cuvier and Brongniart, gave him a surprise performance of *Le Malade Imaginaire*.

These must have been good years, bursting with new ideas and general vitality. At twenty-three he married Madamoiselle Torras, a girl from one of the close-knit Geneva families which had always formed part of his background. From then on he realised that botany was his chosen career.

In 1802 he accepted the task of expanding the *Flore Française* begun by Lamarck, and in the next three years classified and analysed 2,000 new species of plants, in addition to the 2,700 listed by Lamarck. The new addition of *Flore Française* appeared in five volumes in 1805 – the first *flore* of a large country based on the method of natural families. According to the artist Rodolphe Töpffer, between 1806 and 1812 de Candolle carried out a mission for the French Government which involved covering the length and breadth of France to study the botanical and agricultural scene. His subsequent reports were not only confined to these subjects; and more than once he drew attention to the need for better and more enlightened administration.

In 1808 de Candolle was made Director of the Jardin Botanique at Montpellier – a position which did not conflict with his journeys round France. This was a period of reflection and gestation, giving time for the further development of the many ideas he brought from Paris. Before long de Candolle's salon became a focal point for society, and three or four hundred students were attracted to his botanical lectures which for the first time placed emphasis on organography and vegetal physiology. Once a week, it seems, he led a party of two or three hundred pupils out of the town on a botanical forage, happily answering a barrage of questions on every aspect of plants. During these eight years he transformed the Jardin Botanique and, among many other treatises, published his *Théorie élémentaire de la botanique*. This, cutting as it did across many of the views held by his former colleagues in Paris, was a provocative document and caused a considerable stir.

Auguste de la Rive suggests that this quiet life became, in time, somewhat monotonous for a man of his high intelligence. In 1816 he returned to Geneva, where he knew he would find the rounded life of research and social interplay which he needed.

A story is told of a large audience gathering to hear him lecture at the Academy in Geneva. He never appeared, and eventually the people dispersed. At the following lesson, before sitting down, 'Gentlemen,' he said, 'I owe you an apology. I was working; I had forgotten you. But, if my forgetfulness can give you an idea of the charms of Botany, this lesson which did not take place will have been the best in my course.'[2]

De Candolle taught at the Academy until 1835, becoming equally well-known there as a lecturer. 'His office and his herbarium were open to his pupils at all hours of the day; he himself would interrupt his work with a kindness which made them forget the inconvenience they must be causing him.'[3]

It is hardly surprising that such a man should quickly become established at the heart of Genevan intellectual society. Among many others, the de Candolles were closely connected with the Sismondis who lived nearby. Sismondi, who preferred to call himself Italian but whose family were in fact Genevese, was a distinguished historian and champion of the cause of Italian freedom. He was married to Jessie Allen, one of the talented Allen daughters. Jessie was an early feminist and her niece Emma was married to Charles Darwin. The Sismondi house was perpetually crammed with Italian intellectuals seeking refuge in Geneva, and English travellers. It is worth noting that when Florence Nightingale was just eighteen, in 1837, her parents took their daughters to the Continent, stopping in Geneva on the way back from Italy to visit the Sismondis. Florence's mother, Fanny, and Jessie Allen were old friends, and in their house the young Florence entered another world. Cecil Woodham Smith, in *Florence Nightingale*, tells us of her fascination with Sismondi and his cause. Though very small and apparently almost hideous, he overflowed with charm and goodness of heart. At the same time, Florence's father was particularly drawn to de Candolle, who was to be found at the centre of stimulating conversation wherever they went.

During the years in Geneva, de Candolle produced many papers of importance, notably *L'Organographie végétale*, which appeared in 1827, and *La Physiologie végétale*, which followed five years later. By far his most ambitious work, however, was *Prodromus*, described here by Rodolphe Töpffer:

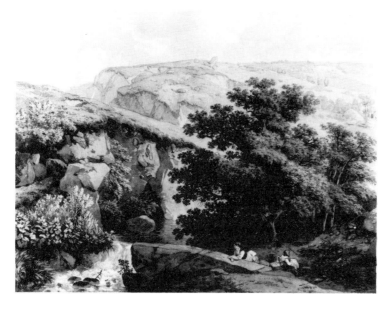

Trees beside a stream in a rocky landscape, with two women looking on, by A. W. Töpffer (*MAH, Geneva; Collection Societé des Arts*)

. . . By slow degrees . . . de Candolle had conceived the gigantic design of publishing a detailed description of all known plants, of examining one by one each species, and of classifying everything according to the then prevailing method. To this end he visited the principal collections of Europe, in order to establish the identity of the synonyms. He undertook this colossal work, and pursued it until the publication of the second volume; but recognising then that, in order to be completed, this undertaking would take no less than 120 years, he shortened the project, and went to work on his *Prodromus systematis regni vegetabilis*, a vast work in itself, since it took sixteen years of incessant labour to publish seven volumes. In these seven volumes half the plants of the globe are described and classified; it is the largest handbook in existence today.[4]

August de la Rive in *Galeries Suisses* notes that such a change of plan was essential on account of the increasing number of plant discoveries being made, thanks to long-distance travellers, now that peace had been restored. When de Candolle began his original work, *le Systema regni végétabilis*, 'the number of known species was from twenty to twenty-five thousand; less than ten

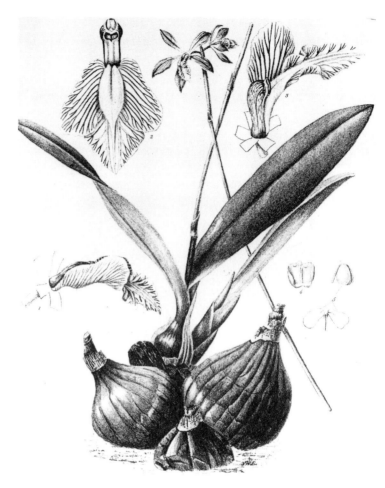

*Epindendrum Candollei
Lindl* 'Having seen this
Epindendrum flower
and having shown it in
Geneva, I took
advantage of a journey
to London to show it to
Dr. Lindley.' (From
*Notes on Rare Plants
cultivated in the
Botanic Garden of
Geneva* by Augustin-
Pyramus and Alphonse
de Candolle)

years later, this figure was doubled; in 1850, it rose to more than a
hundred thousand! . . . in all, in the seven volumes published by
him, he had described six thousand new species.'

One of the seven volumes of *Prodromus* contained the *Flora of
Mexico*. The manner in which these illustrations were copied
from the magnificent collection of a Spanish colleague, as
recounted by Maria Edgeworth to her stepmother, gives clear
indication of de Candolle's reputation.

In September 1840 de Candolle, together with Auguste de la
Rive, took part in a congress at Turin. He was received with
acclamation, but collapsed on the way home. He died a year later,
aged sixty-three, worn out by superhuman output.

De Candolle's contributions to his native town were endless, and in most cases little known. Who, for example, is aware that it was he who was responsible for the erection of Geneva's two iron bridges? Above all, though, the famous Jardin Botanique is his great memorial in the town. Töpffer, in *Magasin Pittoresque*, describes the way in which it was founded:

Having scarcely arrived in Geneva, he makes plans to create a botanical garden. For this, he needs the support of the state; he obtains it . . . he opens a subscription list, which is filled with unbelievable fervour; vases, railings, labels arrive in kind; each citizen, *rentier* or merchant, varnisher or metal-worker, wishes to contribute personally to the project; so well does this charming, dedicated, lively and witty man know how to set alight hearts, and stimulate good intentions . . .'

A man of such international reputation was inevitably linked with other European scientists. De Candolle's son, Alphonse, was also a scientist of distinction, and father and son were in particularly close contact with the English systematists and natural scientists.

In his unpublished notes on *Mémoires et Souvenirs*[5], the elder de Candolle makes various comments on foreigners visiting Geneva. It is interesting, for instance, to read that he returns the compliment where Maria Edgeworth is concerned: '. . . The celebrated Miss Edgeworth, author of very interesting moralistic novels and educational books. She was as simple and good as her works; without having been a great friend of hers, I remember her with affection.' He also writes:

It is not my intention . . . to mention all the travellers I have met since I lived in Geneva, but to say a few words about the most remarkable among them, and about those with whom I have formed close relations. The travellers that I shall mention are of two kinds: the botanists, whom I can without too much presumption believe to have come largely on my account; and people to whom botany is unknown . . .

Amongst the botanists, I will list the following, approximately according to the dates of their visit: . . . *Brown (Robert)* came two or three times to Geneva; in the course of one of his visits he stayed with me. I was very appreciative of his visits, and tried to express to him all the admiration I have for his work and for his character.

Described by J.B. Farmer, in *Makers of British Botany*, as 'the greatest [English] botanist of his day', Robert Brown (1773–1858) was the son of a highly independent-minded clergyman in Montrose, from whom he undoubtedly inherited his strong personality. At the age of twenty-two he joined the Fifeshire regiment of fencibles as surgeon-mate and served six years with them in northern Ireland, where he spent his spare time as an amateur botanist, collecting mosses and liverworts. In 1798 he came to London, where he became an Associate of the Linnean Society and attracted the attention of Sir Joseph Banks. As a result, Sir Joseph offered him the post of naturalist to the *Investigator*, and in 1801 he sailed with Captain Flinders for New Holland. After many adventures he returned to England in 1805, with a collection of 4,000 new plants. These were added to those already brought back by Sir Joseph Banks and other contemporary explorers. In 1805 Brown began the great work of their classification, at the same time becoming librarian to the Linnean Society.

The first volume of his *Prodromus, Florae Novae Hollandae*, published in 1810, owes much to de Candolle – though in it Brown has constructed several new orders, to take account of Australian plants which could not be fitted into de Candolle's smaller list. In the event, only one volume was ever published, but it is in itself an outstanding contribution. It is interesting to note that Brown's *Analysis of the structure of Polygala* 'was adopted by de Candolle . . . in . . . the first volume of his *Prodromus*'.[6]

By 1810 Robert Brown had become the leading systematist of his time in England. In the following year he was made a Fellow of the Royal Society, and the King of Prussia decorated him with the Order *Pour le Mérite*.

At this time he was appointed librarian to Sir Joseph Banks and thereafter became the focal point for collections brought back by travellers from abroad: notably a herbarium collected in Abyssinia in 1805 and 1810, by Henry Salt; and Professor Christian Smith's herbarium, brought back from the Congo in 1816.

Throughout an unusually distinguished life, Brown's personality made a strong impression on all who came in contact with him. He was in fact a very canny Scot when it came to business, as the trustees of the British Museum learned to their cost in connection with the disposal of the Banksian collections.

His connections with the Linnean Society were always close. Sir Joseph Banks left him his house in Soho Square and, as it was larger than he required for his own needs, the Linnean Society occupied a number of rooms for some years. In 1840 he became its president. This great botanist eventually died in his eighty-fifth year – mentally alert and interested in his ruling passion to the end.

De Candolle's son, Alphonse, editor of the *Mémoires et Souvenirs*, noted:

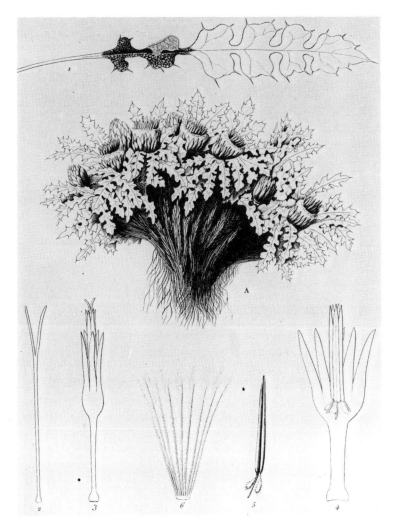

Aplotaxis leontodontoides (From *Memoir on the Structure and Classification of the 'Composées' Family* by Augustin-Pyramus de Candolle)

Having often had the opportunity to see Monsieur Robert
Brown, who was very good to me, I am sure that he was as
attached to my father as my father was to him; but one must
admit that the differences in their characters and their
behaviour was at times laughable. One day, in particular,
Brown arrived without warning in Geneva at my father's
office. The latter was so surprised and delighted that, giving
way to the demonstrative emotions inherited from his
meridional origins and 're-charged' at Montpellier, he threw
himself on Brown's neck. Never did an Englishman pull a
more piteous face in a similar situation . . . I was extremely
amused.

On a visit to Brown in London in 1826, Alphonse de Candolle
sent his father an account of how Brown took him to the Linnean
Society, where they elected as president Lord Stanley, son of
Lord Derby. He described the dinner which followed and the
discussions which took place concerning the future of Linnaeus's
herbarium.

The President turned towards me during one of his
discussions saying that he asked the foreigners to forgive him
but that he very much wanted Linnaeus's herbarium to
remain in England. They looked at me laughing, and I made
a sign to them of approval so that they would not believe you
wanted to take it away from them.[7]

Continuing his reminiscences of distinguished botanists, the
elder de Candolle mentioned George Bentham:

Bentham, nephew of the celebrated Jeremy, came several
times to Geneva. He is an outstanding botanist, exact and
hard-working, and what is more an excellent man, for whose
friendship I have a real attachment. He has done me many
little services relative to science; he has been very kind to my
son during his journeys in England. Part of his youth having
been passed at Montpellier since my departure, he had so
often heard me spoken of that we found, so to speak, that we
were linked in friendship before we had met.[8]

Alphonse de Candolle, his son, added the following lines:
'Monsieur George Bentham told me and wrote again and again

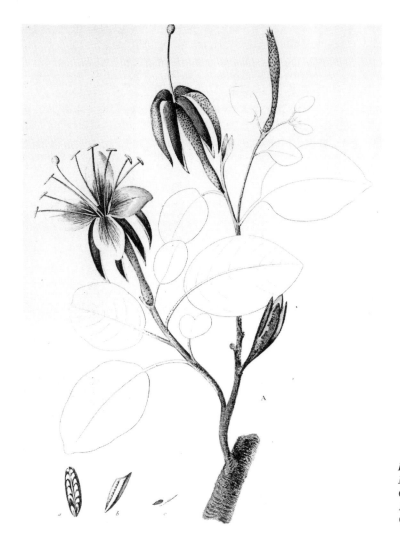

Hauya elegans (From *Memoir on the Onagraites Family* by Augustin-Pyramus de Candolle)

that he regarded himself as one of my father's pupils. He acquired his taste for botany through *La Flore Française*.'

George Bentham (1800–1884) was born into an unusually gifted family. His father, Sir Samuel Bentham, was an inspector of dockyards, while his mother was intellectual and energetic. All the children were clever. When George was five, the family went to Russia for two years, as his father was on a mission to St Petersburg. The children received a firm grounding in Russian, French and German during these two years. On the return voyage, bad weather forced them to spend some weeks in Sweden and, of course, George and his siblings quickly learned Swedish.

For the next seven years the family lived in England and the children were privately taught by tutors. Thereafter, the family moved to France, where they remained till 1827. Writing in his diary from Paris, George describes the people he was meeting with his family, including Walter Savage Landor, Talleyrand and Humbold. Humbold gave him great encouragement in his studies of physical geography. On a tour with the family in France, George found a copy of de Candolle's *Flore Française* in an Angoulême hotel. It so excited him that he picked up a flower in the small garden behind the house and proceeded to analyse it, succeeding in assigning it to its right species.

The family spent some months at Montauban, and George became a student at the faculty of theology there, studying, amongst other subjects, botany. His father had evidently acquired a large estate near Montpellier and, on the death of his elder brother, George became its manager. It was at this time that he translated into French his uncle Jeremy Bentham's chapters on nomenclature and classification from the *Chrestomathia*, amplifying considerably the portions relating to the arts and sciences. This was published in Paris in 1823, and it established George Bentham's position in France as an acute analyser, clear expositor and cautious reasoner.

His next few years were thoroughly frustrating, in that his uncle insisted on his constant help, at a time when he himself was trying to study law. Worse, he was called upon to put in order his father's vast output of writings on the navy and dockyards. He had to give up his law studies, and had no time to pursue his botanical research. However, father and uncle died within a year of each other, in 1831–2, and at last he found himself free.

He was elected a fellow of the Linnean Society in 1828, and Robert Brown proposed him for the Royal Society in 1829. On Brown's recommendation, however, he, as well as other scientific candidates, withdrew in protest at the election of a royal duke as President of the Society. Before long, as a result of prolonged travel, Bentham was in close contact with the great figures of natural classification – de Candolle, Brown, Enlicher, Lindley and Hooker.

From 1829–40 he was honorary secretary to the Horticultural Society. This was a time when travellers were bringing back a whole series of unknown plants, and these were carefully named and described by Bentham and Lindley, the assistant secretary.

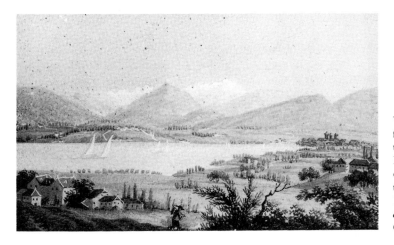

View of Lake Geneva, flanked by the Salève, the Môle and the Mont Blanc range; miniature on a musical-box, from the Genevese School *c.* 1850 (*Collection Musée d'art et d'histoire, Geneva*)

In particular, Dr Wallich's presentation of the East India Company's marvellous collection afforded them important material to work on.

In 1834 Bentham, who married the daughter of the former British Ambassador to Persia, Sir Harford Brydges, moved first to his uncle's house in Queen Square Place, London, and later to Pontrian House, Hereford, where he was better able to accommodate his vast herbarium and library. In 1854 he handed over the latter to Kew Gardens, and Sir William Hooker, hearing of his intention to give up botany, prevailed on him to keep a room at Kew and lend them his co-operation with a new series on colonial flora. He became President of the Linnean Society in 1861, and continued to run the Society for the next thirteen years.

Bentham's greatest contribution was his major share in the *Genera Plantarum*. Sir Joseph Hooker was responsible for the remaining section and the work took more than twenty-five years.

> The Candollean arrangement of orders is maintained for the most part, but nearly every important order is remodelled. Such a work marks of necessity an epoch in botany, and Bentham's share in it is his most enduring monument.

He died a year after its conclusion, at the age of eighty-four.

Another English scientist with whom de Candolle was linked was Sir Humphry Davy (1778–1829), inventor of the Davy Lamp.

In 1813, despite the war between England and France, Davy

succeeded in obtaining permission from Napoleon to visit Paris. He had by then received European acclaim and had been awarded the Napoleon Prize by the Institut de France. From Paris he travelled to Montpellier, where he stayed some time with de Candolle. The two men were very different in temperament, which precluded real intimacy between them, but each had great admiration for the other.

The following autumn Davy went abroad with his wife, taking with him Michael Faraday,[9] who was at that time a young assistant in the Royal Institution laboratory. They went first to

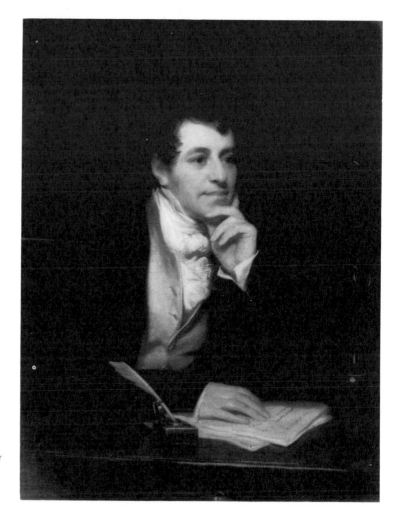

Sir Humphry Davy, by T. Phillips (*National Portrait Gallery, London*)

Paris, and thence to Italy. On the way back they stopped in Geneva. De Candolle was still living in Montpellier, and they dined with the Marcets. (It will be remembered that Jane Marcet, née Haldimand, was the authoress with whom Maria Edgeworth corresponded for many years.)

Roger de Candolle, Augustin-Pyramus' surviving male descendant, relates the following anecdote about the evening. It appears that when dinner was announced Madame Marcet was about to lead the way into the dining-room when Lady Davy (who, as a very powerful widow, had only recently become Sir Humphry's wife) said loudly, 'Mr Faraday, you will now go and eat your meal in the kitchen!' The unfortunate Faraday vanished below stairs while the rest of the party seated themselves at table. At the end of dinner, when the ladies rose to leave the gentlemen, their host was heard to remark in a loud whisper, 'And now, my dear Sirs, let us go and join Mr Faraday in the kitchen!'

Six years earlier, Davy had been elected as secretary of the Royal Society, subsequently becoming a member of the Council. In 1816 de Candolle visited London, and in letters to his family spoke of seeing and spending time with Davy. In 1820 Davy was made president of the Royal Society, in succession to Sir Joseph Banks. His health, however, was beginning to fail and, recuperating in Italy, he wrote to the Royal Society declaring his wish to resign from the Presidency.[10]

He returned to England in October 1827, but left again for Italy a few months later. In March 1829 he wrote to his brother from Rome saying he was dying. However, he rallied, and travelled by slow stages to Geneva, which he reached on 28 May. He died half a day later and was buried in the cemetery of Plain-Palais. De Candolle made an outstanding eulogy at the funeral.

Among the most distinguished of de Candolle's colleagues were William and Joseph Hooker of Kew, father and son. Roger de Candolle, referring to the ties between Augustin-Pyramus and Alphonse on the one side and William and Joseph on the other, writes:

Apart from the numerous references in family correspondence, the de Candolle Foundation has fourteen letters from Sir William to Augustin Pyramus dating from 1816 to 1833 and eighteen letters of the same to Alphonse dating from 1828 to 1858. There are also sixty-six letters from Sir Joseph to Alphonse, dated 1845 to 1881 all of which but twelve are not of a personal nature and therefore are at the Conservatoire de Botanique. As for meetings between them, *Mémoires et Souvenirs* makes the following reference to William in 1814: 'Hooker, the English botanist, who came to stay with me for three days, whom I took herborising in this country which was quite new to him (Montpellier), and with whom I have preserved friendly relations . . .'

After this visit Jacob de Candolle, Augustin-Pyramus' banker brother, writes to him from Geneva on 22 June 1814 that Hooker had arrived in Geneva and 'has been well received by all. He has seen Jurine, De Luc, . . . each one wants to give him plants . . . He is dining here this evening.'

During his visit to London in 1816, de Candolle says that he went to see Hooker at Halesworth and that 'this visit although very rapid had for me much interest. He received me with a great deal of friendship and I stayed several days with him. Madame is very charming.' He visits his [Hooker's] herbarium and his small garden. There he also meets his pupil Lindley. In 1819 he again sees him in London.

In 1838 a letter from Augustin-Pyramus to Alphonse who is in England recommends that he should see 'the good Hooker', and talks about exchanging plants with him. In August of that year Alphonse is in Glasgow and stays with William.[11]

Between them, the Hookers administered Kew for more than forty years. William Hooker (1785–1865) was elected to the Linnean Society at the age of twenty-one and, amongst other natural historians of the time, got to know Robert Brown and Sir Joseph Banks.

He had already penetrated into the innermost circle of the Science of the country. For a period of sixty years he held there a place unique in its activity. He shared with Augustin-Pyramus de Candolle and with Robert Brown the position of greatest prominence amongst systematists . . . The interval between the death of Linnaeus and the publication of the *Origin of Species* can show no greater triumvirate of botanists than these, working each in his own way, but simultaneously.[14]

William Hooker's outstanding offices were the Regius Chair of

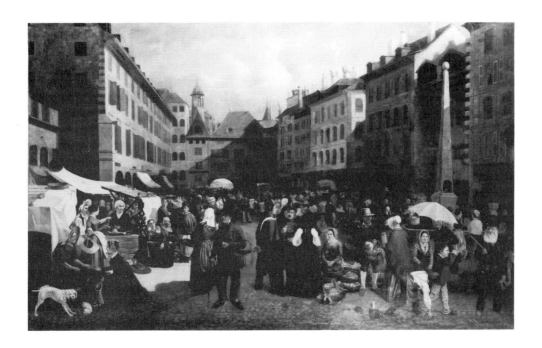

Botany in Glasgow (1820–41) and Director of Kew Gardens (1841–65). In 1800 he visited Iceland, but, disastrously, the collection he made there – above all the cryptogams – was destroyed when his ship caught fire on the journey home. In 1814, he went to France to meet the leading botanists there. This was the occasion when he visited de Candolle at Montpellier and went 'herborising' with him.

La Place du Molard in 1843 by Henri-Germain Lacombe (*Collection Musée d'art et d'histoire, Geneva*)

He was offered the Chair in Botany at Glasgow University in 1820, and on his arrival there immediately set about improving and extending the newly-opened botanic garden. There was enormous public enthusiasm for the project, and before long – due largely to William Hooker's own efforts – plants began to arrive from all parts of the globe. Gradually connections were built up with other botanical gardens, many of them world-wide.

Hooker had never lectured before, but it appears that his courses, though unorthodox, were highly successful, and for the first time incorporated field-work. When he went to Kew, he took with him, of course, his herbarium and his library. Kew was at a low point when he reached it and, in the years that followed, he built up the garden to be not only a national centre but a source of knowledge for the Empire, and indeed for the whole world. His

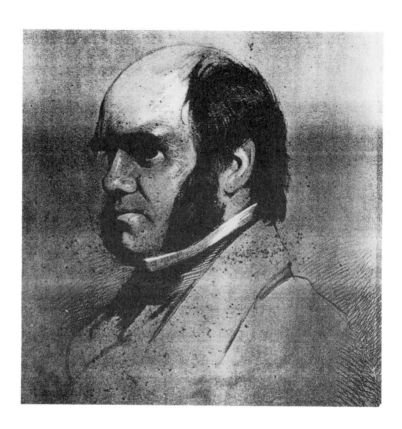

Darwin in 1853, by
Samuel Lawrence

herbarium and library were at first lodged in his own house. However, in 1853 he moved into the official residence, and they were transferred to a place in the botanic garden and made available to visiting botanists. George Bentham's enormous herbarium and library were added to this collection in 1857.

When his father died in 1865, Joseph Hooker (1817–1911) succeeded him as director at Kew and continued the work of administration. His extensive and prolific travels began when he was twenty-two and sailed as assistant surgeon and botanist in the *Erebus* and then the *Terror*. For four years the captain, James Ross, led his ships on what was, in effect, a magnetic survey of the Antarctic. This resulted in Joseph Hooker's first scientific work, *The Antarctic Flora*.

Before leaving for the Antarctic, Joseph had met Charles Darwin, briefly but agreeably, in Trafalgar Square.

In January 1844 Hooker received the memorable letter

confiding to him the germ of the Theory of Descent. Darwin wrote this: 'At last gleams of light have come, and I am almost convinced that species are not (it is like confessing a murder) immutable: I think I have found (here's presumption!) the simple way by which species become exquisitely adapted to various ends.'[12]

Joseph's subsequent prolific travels – in the Himalayas, the Middle East, the Atlas Mountains and, in old age, the Rocky Mountains – yielded findings which substantially contributed to the 'origin of species', and Darwin wrote to him in 1845: 'I know I shall live to see you the first authority in Europe on that grand subject, that almost keystone of the laws of Creation, Geographic Distribution.'[13]

A strong friendship developed between Darwin and Hooker. Soon after he and Wallace had given their great exposé to the Linnean Society, Darwin wrote to his associate: 'Dr Hooker has become almost as heterodox as you or I; and I look at Hooker as by far the most capable judge in Europe.'[14]

A series of essays, beginning with the introductory essay to the *Flora Tasmaniae* (which in fact covered the *Antarctic Flora* as a whole), gave Joseph Hooker in his day his reputation as 'philosophical biologist', and in our time mark him out as the first ecologist. They were the result of long and careful thought and analysis and, by the process of what Darwin referred to as his own 'self-thought', Hooker arrived eventually at 'the hypothesis that species are derivative, and mutable.'

They were a rare breed of men – de Candolle and his friends and colleagues. Drawn from widely differing backgrounds, with the exception of Davy they all shared the same systematic approach to botany, and all were caught up in the euphoria of eighteenth- and nineteenth-century scientific discovery. From what can be gathered, all were genial, gifted men, and all, apart from de Candolle, lived to ripe and useful old age. As for de Candolle himself, he emerges not only as a brilliantly gifted scientist but also as an exceptional human being. This wise and most cultivated man brought warmth to all his relationships, loved his family, enjoyed society (not least the company of charming and intelligent women) and was proud of his Genevan roots. He would be a great man in any age.

Although Joseph Hooker never met de Candolle, the blazing of the trail which led from Linnaeus to Darwin and his own contribution to geographic distribution was accomplished thanks

to the dedication of de Candolle, Brown, and Joseph Hooker's
father William, who worked patiently and logically to piece
together the systematist pattern.

Notes

1. *A-P de Candolle*, Auguste de la Rive, Paris 1851. De la Rive was
   a distinguished natural scientist and, among many other honours
   conferred on him, an Associate of the Royal Society, London.
2. *Galeries Suisses*, Felix Bungener, article in 'Biographies
   Nationales'.
3. *A-P de Candolle*, Auguste de la Rive, Paris, 1851.
4. *Magasin Pittoresque*, Rodolphe Töpffer; quoted by de la Rive in
   Galeries Suisses.
5. In the possession of the Fondation Augustin-Pyramus de
   Candolle.
6. *Makers of British Botany*, J.B. Farmer, edited by R.W. Oliver.
7. *Catalogue Raisonne des Lettres d'Alphonse de Candolle*, in
   possession of the Fondation Augustin-Pyramus de Candolle.
8. *Mémoires et Souvenirs*, in the possession of the Fondation
   Augustin-Pyramus de Candolle.
9. Michael Faraday, the inventor of electricity.
10. Davy contributed forty-six memoirs and lectures to the
    transactions of the Royal Society, and he published nine separate
    works on science.
11. Extract from letter to the author from Roger de Candolle,
    October 1985.
12. *Makers of British Botany*, F.O. Bower, edited by R.W. Oliver.
13. Ibid.
14. Ibid.

CHAPTER 5

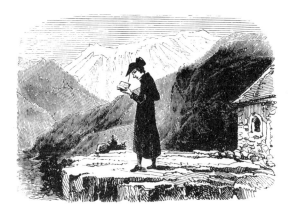

LITERARY VISITORS

In 1824, Frederick Gye, a very unpoetical but prosperous Englishman taking his family on the Grand Tour, arrived at the Hotel d'Angleterre at Sécheron and noted peevishly in his diary:

> *Tuesday, September 27th*: . . . Before 9a.m. we reached the Hôtel d'Angleterre at Geneva, or rather at a place called Sécheron. . . . Geneva is a large place, of remarkable architecture, with very little worthy of notice about it, if one excepts the Lake, which is certainly very fine . . . We strolled through the town several hours, and as it is said to be remarkable for Jewellery, we particularly noticed those shops: they are miserable little dwellings, with little glass cases put out at their doors, to shew their goods, and there is not even one that if in London we should call even a decent shop . . . Returned to Hotel, and dined at six. Champagne not drinkable. Tried a second bottle; sent that away also. Retired early . . . September 30th: Breakfasted at nine, and paid most extravagant bill we had yet had – six francs a head for dinner, and they charged the bad champagne.[1]

Monsieur Dejean, proprietor of the Hôtel d'Angleterre at Sécheron, was, however, a remarkable businessman. Any landlord capable of organising a fleet of thirty-five calèches to be ready at Calais to transport those Englishmen embarking on the Grand Tour across Europe to Lake Geneva and his own hotel deserves admiration. In addition to a host of distinguished and less distinguished English visitors, he had entertained both the

Empress Josephine and Queen Hortense. In short, his hotel was generally considered to be comfortable, clean and well-placed.

Eight years prior to the visit of Francis Gye, on 25 March 1816, Lord Byron had arrived at the Hôtel d'Angleterre and in signing the register had given his age as '100', to the annoyance of Dejean. This brilliant, moody, sometimes violent young man had been forced by public opinion to leave England indefinitely. Society had for long been amused by the clashing facets in the Byron character. Recently, however, two factors had come to light which were discussed in every drawing-room: the incestuous relationship between Byron and his half-sister Augusta (in which he appeared to glory), and his sadistic treatment of Lady Byron, the former Annabella Milbanke. In a society where superficial morality provided a screen for venal indulgence, this went far beyond the accepted pattern, and its members rose almost to a man and ostracised him.

Percy Bysshe Shelley, Mary Godwin and her half-sister Claire had already been at Sécheron twelve days. Claire, who had forced Byron to seduce her before leaving London (using the double lure of an introduction to Shelley, whom she knew Byron longed to meet, and to Mary, daughter of Mary Wollstonecraft), had carefully contrived a meeting at the Hôtel d'Angleterre.

Byron's travelling companion was a young Scottish doctor, John Polidori, who had literary aspirations. The publisher Murray had promised him £500 for the manuscript of a diary covering their journey. Shortly after their arrival at Sécheron, he wrote:

> Percy Shelley, author of *Queen Mab*, came: beautiful, shy, consumptive, twenty-one [he was twenty-three]; separated from his wife; keeps the two daughters of Godwin, who practise his theories; one Lord Byron's.

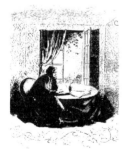

Rodolphe Töpffer chronicling his *Nouveaux Voyages en Zigzag*

The two men were instantly drawn to one another and spent hours every day rowing on the lake. Before long, Shelley leased a cottage across the lake – at Montalègre, near Cologny. Soon after, Byron moved into the Villa Diodati nearby. Their departure was viewed with chagrin by Dejean, for people had been flocking from Geneva to catch a glimpse of the notorious English Milord and business at the Hotel d'Angleterre had been unusually brisk. However, nothing daunted, he promptly installed a telescope on the terrace, and for a consideration visitors were able to turn it on to the Villa Diodati, in the hope of catching a glimpse of what they sought.

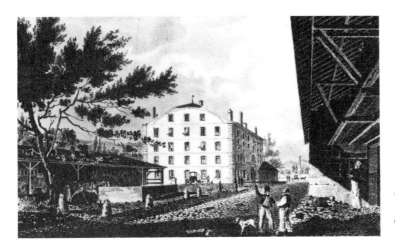

L'auberge of Sécheron, early nineteenth century (*Bibliothèque Publique et Universitaire, Geneva*)

An agreeable pattern of life was soon established between the two households. Days were spent out in the boat and as often as not they all gathered in the evening at the Villa Diodati. Byron was drawn by admiration to Shelley. Each seemed to complement the other: Shelley with his vivid intelligence, shrill accents and pantheistic beliefs; Byron sombrely but uncertainly aware of the powers of God and the Devil: Shelley a pure being; Byron a model for the Don Juan of his creation. They talked endlessly and quickly became inseparable.

Their subsequent tour of the lake in Shelley's boat left its mark on both of them. They revelled in Rousseau's *Meillerie*, wandering, book in hand, as they declaimed the *Nouvelle Héloise*. The castle at Chillon moved Byron to write his famous *Prisoner of Chillon* which, we are told, he composed in one night. And, as the waves lapped against their boat, Shelley conceived his *Hymn to Intellectual Beauty* while Byron added more verses to *Childe Harold*. Each stimulated the other to intellectual achievement. And yet, how astonishingly different they were! Shelley succeeded in conveying to Byron an appreciation of Wordsworth, whose poetry Byron had hitherto shunned. He became for the first time susceptible to the beauty and power of nature, and his verse at this period is clearly Wordsworth-influenced.

Towards the end of July, Shelley, Mary and Claire went off to explore Chamonix and Mont Blanc. At the various hotels where they stayed, Shelley wrote, beneath his name in the visitors' book: 'Democratic, most philanthropic, and godless'.

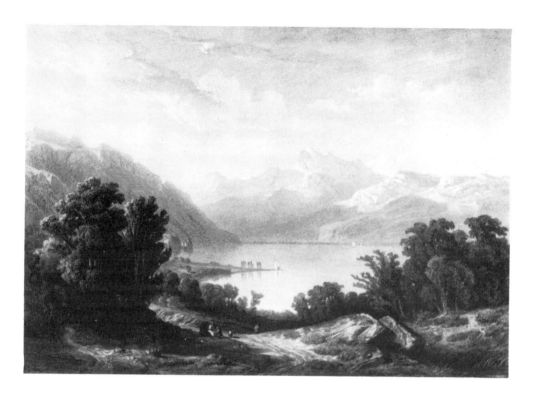

View of the Château of Chillon and the Dents du Midi, by François Diday (*MAH, Geneva; Collection Societé des Arts*)

When Byron passed that way a month later, with his friends Hobhouse and Scrope Davies, he carefully erased the phrase when he saw it in their hotel at Sallanches, saying: 'Do you not think I should do Shelley a service by scratching this out?'

Shelley and his companions were away six days, and at Chamonix saw the *Mer de Glace*, the *Source of the Aveyron*, and the *Glacier de Bosson*. In a letter to his friend Peacock, Shelley described their journey, without, however, telling him of the poem he had written on Mont Blanc, which in fact incorporated many of the phrases he used in the letter:

> . . . Some say that gleams of a remoter world
> Visit the soul in sleep, – that death is slumber,
> And that its shapes the busy thoughts outnumber
> Of those who wake and live. I look on high;
> Has some unknown omnipotence unfurled
> The veil of life and death? Or do I lie
> In dream, and does the mightier world of sleep
> Spread far around and inaccessibly

Its circles? for the very spirit faie,
Driven like a homeless cloud from step to steep
That vanishes among the viewless gales!
Far, far above, piercing the infinite sky,
Mont Blanc appears – still, snowy, and serene.
Its subject mountains their unearthly forms
Pile around it, ice and rock; broad vales between
Of frozen floods, unfathomable deeps,
Blue as the overhanging heaven, that spread
And wind among the accumulated steeps;
A desert peopled by the storms alone,
Save when the eagle brings some hunter's bone,
And the wolf tracks her there [. . .]

Remote, serene, and inaccessible;
And *this* the naked countenance of earth
On which I gaze, even these primaeval mountains,
Teach the adverting mind. The glaciers creep,
Like snakes that watch their prey, from their far fountains,
Slow rolling on . . .

Meanwhile, Byron had fallen into the habit of visiting Madame de Staël at Coppet. He appears to have had a sort of love-hate relationship with her – regarding her as the 'cleverest woman he had ever met', enjoying her wit, yet finding her singularly charmless.

The story of his first visit is apocryphal. On hearing his name announced to the guests, a certain Mrs Hervey (sister of William Beckford) fell into a dead faint. Whereupon Madame de Staël's daughter, the lovely duchesse de Broglie, remarked: 'this is *too much* – at 65 years of age'. As for Germaine de Staël herself, it unquestionably pleased her to have the notorious Byron under her roof. 'Byron, whom nobody else receives except me, is nevertheless the man who occupies everyone most,' she wrote, though with some inaccuracy. Byron had in fact received several friendly overtures from Geneva society when he first arrived at Sécheron. Charles Hentsch, the banker, was an early caller at the Hôtel d'Angleterre, and it seems that Byron saw him frequently while in the vicinity of Geneva. Marc-Auguste Pictet also called. He persuaded Byron to accompany him to a soirée at the home of his cousin Madame Eynard, and here he met Charles-Victor de Bonstetten, who charmed him. In fact, if the truth were told, it was not so much a matter of Byron being snubbed by local society

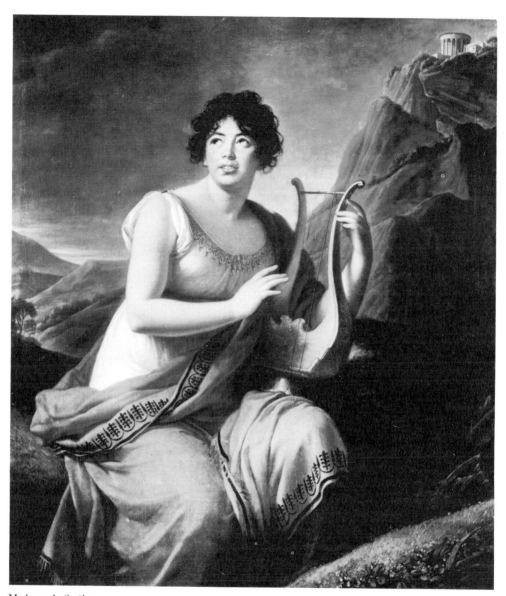

Madame de Staël as
'Corinne' by Elisabeth-
Louise Vigée-Lebrun
(*Collection Musée d'art
et d'histoire, Geneva*)

as local society being held at arm's length by Byron. And while there was a chance of spending hours and days with Shelley, he wished to look no further.

Now, however, he rather relished sparring with Madame de Staël at Coppet, enjoying the stimulation of her scolding. 'You ought not to have taken on the world,' she is reported to have said to him. 'It's an impossibility. The world is too strong for an individual. I tried it myself when I was young – but it's impossible.'

This period has been referred to as the 'Indian Summer' of Coppet. In *Mistress to an Age*, Christopher Herold refers to

> Delicate and Secret negotiations, carried on against a background of feasts and talk. Among the guests Byron met at Coppet were Lord Lansdowne, Henry Brougham, Pellegrino Rossi, Etienne Dumont, Sismondi, several score of dukes and princes, English and Continental, and every liberal in Geneva. 'She has made Coppet as agreeable as society and talent can make any place on earth,' said Byron.

Madame de Staël was sympathetic on the subject of Lady Byron, and Byron accepted her offer to mediate between them. Alas, not even she could work such a miracle; and it could be argued that Germaine de Staël would scarcely be the 'go-between' acceptable to the morally-outraged Annabella.

On 29 August, Shelley, Mary and Claire left for England. The same day, Byron set out for Chamonix, taking with him Scrope Davies and Hobhouse, who were his guests at the Villa Diodati. A little later on, he and Hobhouse visited the Bernese Oberland. (Before doing so, he dismissed the hapless Polidori, whose insufferable vanity and literary pretensions had irritated all of them for so long.) Shelley's influence was still strong, and the general effect produced by the elemental grandeur of the Alps undoubtedly helped nurture *Manfred*:[2]

Voice of the SECOND SPIRIT[3]

> Mont Blanc is the monarch of mountains;
>   They crown'd him long ago
> On a throne of rocks, in a robe of clouds,
>   With a diadem of snow,
> Around his waist are forests braced,
>   The Avalanche in his hand;

> But ere it fall, that thundering ball
>   Must pause for my command.
> The Glacier's cold and restless mass
>   Moves onward day by day;
> But I am he who bids it pass,
>   Or with its ice delay.
> I am the spirit of the place,
>   Could make the mountain bow
> And quiver to his cavern'd base –
>   And what with me would'st *Thou*?

Matthew (Monk) Lewis had recently visited Byron, and while at the Diodati had translated some of Goethe's *Faust* for him. To the brooding, desperate Byron, constantly preoccupied with the diabolic, the theme had the most powerful appeal. He began *Manfred* while still on his travels, and into it poured all his reactions to elemental landscape, all his personal despair. Astarte is Augusta; he (Byron), *Manfred*; and the being addressed in the terrifying magic chant, Annabella. It is all there. Although the word 'incest' is never spoken, it appears implicitly in the poem, and Byron's fearful remorse is exposed for all to read. To Tom Moore he wrote, 'I was half mad between metaphysics, mountains, lakes, love unextinguishable, thoughts unutterable, and the nightmare of my own delinquencies.'

Autumn had descended on Geneva and the lake. Shelley had left, Coppet was emptying, and it was time for Byron too to move on. He left Diodati on 5 October, and with Hobhouse took the road to Milan, using the Simplon Pass.

John Ruskin was from childhood emotionally involved with Geneva. His life was changed when, on his thirteenth birthday on 8 February 1832, his father's business partner introduced him to Turner's drawings and water-colours. In 1833, Prout's book of sketches in Flanders and Germany decided the family to take their annual holiday in Germany and Switzerland, with the hope of continuing to Rome. In the event, the heat deflected them to Geneva and Chamonix, where Ruskin's love-affair with both places began. Of Geneva he writes:

> . . . A little canton four miles square, and which did not wish to be six miles square! A little town, composed of a cluster of water-mills, a street of penthouses, two wooden bridges, two dozen of stone houses on a little hill, and three or four

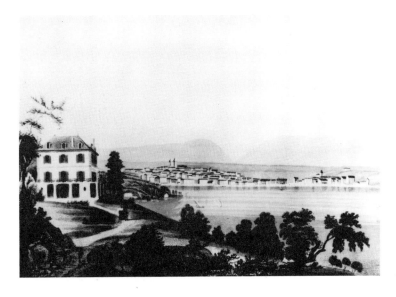

Villa Diodati, *c*. 1820
(*Photograph: François Martin*)

perpendicular lanes up and down the hill. The four miles of
acreage round, in grass, with modest gardens, and farm-
dwelling houses; the people, pious, learned, and busy, to a
man, to a woman – to a boy, to a girl of them; progressing to
and fro mostly on their feet, and only where they had
business. And this bird's nest of a place, to be the centre of
religious and social thought, and of physical beauty, to all
living Europe! . . . this inconceivable point of patience.[4]

Ruskin's upbringing was in a typical industrial middle-class,
virtuous Victorian family, living in Croydon, outside London.

. . . Mrs Ruskin would not let John play with his Croydon
cousins because their father was a baker who lived over the
shop . . . The social graces were entirely absent, and with
them the whole concept of taste.[5]

'The reader must have felt,' says Ruskin, 'that, though very
respectable people in our way, we were all of us definitely vulgar
people, just as my aunt's dog, Towzer, was a vulgar dog, though a
very good and dear dog. Said reader should have seen also that we
had not set ourselves up to have a taste in anything.'[6]

Ruskin's childhood and adolescence were plagued by sickness,
and in time this led to frequent return-visits to Geneva. In the

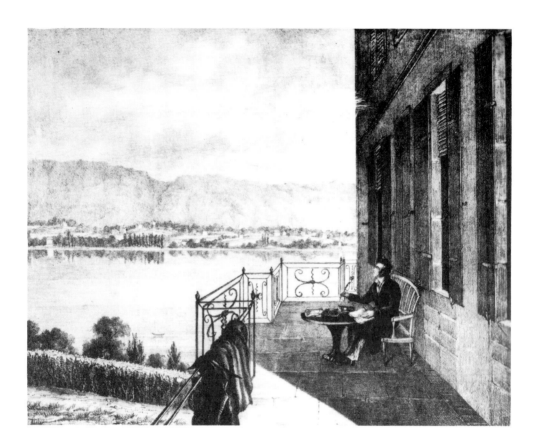

Lord Byron on the
terrace at the Villa
Diodati, 1816:
(*Bibliothèque Publique
et Universitaire,
Geneva*)

Praeterita, he gives us a detailed account of the often-repeated
journey through Paris, Dijon, and finally the mountainous Juras –
before the climactic arrival at the Col de la Faucille:

> . . . [the road ascends] very slightly . . . and a sweep of the
> road, traversed in five minutes at a trot, opens the whole
> Lake of Geneva, and the chain of the Alps along 100 miles of
> horizon . . .

In discussion of an early journey, Ruskin tells us 'there have
been, in sum, three centres of my life's thought: Rouen, Geneva
and Pisa . . . [they] have been tutresses of all I know, and were
mistresses of all I did, from the first moments I entered their
gates.' And later, he writes; 'Of my early joy in Milan, I have
already told; of Geneva there is no telling.'

Ruskin is at all times absorbed by the river Rhône:

... For all other rivers there is a surface, and an underneath, and a vaguely displeasing idea of the bottom. But the Rhône flows like one lambent jewel; its surface is nowhere, its ethereal self is everywhere, the irridescent rush and translucent strength of it blue to the shore, and radiant to the depth. Fifteen feet thick, of not flowing, but flying water; not water, neither, – melted glacier, rather, one should call it; the force of the ice is with it, and the wreathing of the clouds, the gladness of the sky, and the continuance of Time ...

As for Chamonix, it fascinated him from the beginning, and in June 1844, his father placed him in the care of Joseph Couttet, the captain of Mont Blanc, then in his sixtieth year: 'For thirty years he remained my tutor and companion. Had he been my drawing-master also, it would have been better for me: if my work pleased Couttet, it was always good.'

Ruskin, throughout his life, had the tenderest health, and there is no doubt that the very air of Geneva and Mont Blanc had a therapeutic effect on him. Geneva and Chamonix were a life-line of beauty and sanity for him; he was constantly reaching for them.

George Eliot (Miss Evans) was born in 1821 – two years after Ruskin. The exceptionally gifted daughter of a wealthy farmer and estate agent, she grew up in a small Warwickshire village, moving at the age of twenty-one with her widowed father to Coventry. Although plagued by migraine and backache, she settled down to a quiet but intellectually stimulating life, reading voraciously and translating Strauss's *Leben Jesu*. Her father's health, however, began to deteriorate, and she nursed him devotedly through his last long illness. Over-strained as she was, his death at the end of May 1849 devastated her and she became deeply depressed.

A year or so before, writing to John Sibree, the brother of a friend, who the following year published a translation of Hegel's lectures on the *Philosophy of History*, she told him: 'I like the notion of your going to Germany as good in every way for yourself, body and mind, and for all others. Oh the bliss of having a very high attic in a romantic Continental town, such as Geneva – far away from morning callers, dinners and decencies, and then to pause for a year and think *de omnibus rebus et quibusdam aliis*, and then to return to life, and work for poor stricken humanity, and never think of self again!'

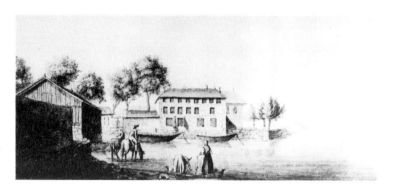

The Quai de Paquis,
early nineteenth century
(*Photograph: François
Martin*)

Now it seemed she would realise this wish. Fortunately, her
admirable and devoted friends the Bray-Hennells from Coventry
were on the point of leaving for the Continent, and insisted on her
going with them. After travelling through France and Italy, they
arrived in Geneva in the third week of July, and George Eliot
decided to remain there when the time came for the party to
return to England.

For the next six months George Eliot lived happily in two
pensions in Geneva – first at the Campagne Plongeon, 'which
stands on a slight eminence a few hundred yards back from the
road on the route d'Hermance', and later, in the rue des
Chanoines, with Monsieur and Madame d'Albert Durade. Despite

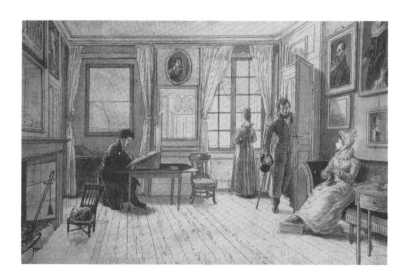

A Genevese Family,
showing a young boy
drawing at his desk,
Genevese School, *c.*
1820 (*Cabinet des
Dessins, Collection
Musée d'art et
d'histoire, Geneva*)

recurring *malaises*, she was gently happy at the Campagne Plongeon, where she was made much of by fellow guests.

> . . . I feel perfectly at home. This place looks more lovely to me every day – The Lake, the town, the *campagnes* with their stately trees and pretty houses, the glorious mountains in the distance; one can hardly believe one's self on earth; one might live here and forget that there is such a thing as want or labour or sorrow.

107, rue des Chanoines, however, was something else. In *George Eliot's Life, as related in her Letters and Journals,* arranged and edited by her husband, J.W. Cross, he wrote in 1885 that No. 107 had become No. 18 and was occupied as the printing-office of the *Journal de Genève*. From the moment she arrived there, George Eliot loved the d'Alberts. Monsieur d'Albert was 'an artist of great respectability', 'Monsieur and Madame d'Albert are middle-aged – musical, and, I am told, have *beaucoup d'esprit*.' And soon after: 'M. and Mme. d'Albert are really clever people – people worth sitting up an hour longer to talk to . . . M. d'Albert plays and sings, and in the winter he tells me they have parties to sing masses and do other delightful things. In fact, I think I am just in the right place.'

On 28 October, she writes to the Brays:

> . . . We have had some delicious autumn days here. If the fine weather lasts, I am going up the Salève on Sunday with Monsieur d'Albert. . . . The walks about Geneva are perfectly enchanting. . . .
>
> . . . I like my town life vastly . . . There is an indescribable charm to me in this form of human nest-making. You enter a by no means attractive-looking house, you climb up two or three flights of cold, dark-looking stone steps, you ring at a very modest door, and you enter a set of rooms snug, or comfortable, or elegant . . . I have always had a hankering for this sort of life, and I find it was a true instinct of what would suit me. Just opposite my windows is the street in which the Sisters of Charity live . . .

And in a letter dated 4 December:

> My good friends here only change for the better. Madame d'Albert is all affection; Monsieur d'Albert all delicacy and

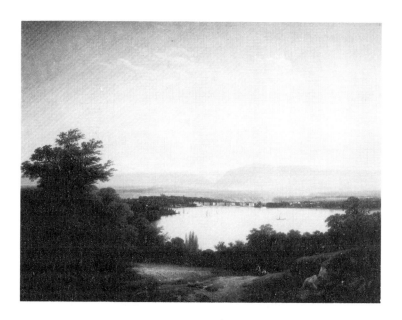

Geneva from Cologny,
by François Diday, *c.*
1845 (*Collection Musée
d'art et d'histoire,
Geneva*)

intelligence; the friends to whom they have introduced me
very kind in their attentions . . . I can say anything to
Monsieur and Madame d'Albert. Monsieur d'Albert
understands everything, and if Madame does not
understand, she believes – that is, she seems always sure that
I mean something edifying. She kisses me like a mother.

Writing on 23 December 1849, Eliot mentions that she is
'attending a course of lectures on Experimental Physics by
Monsieur le Professeur de la Rive, the inventor, amongst other
things, of the electro-plating'. And then later: 'We have had Alboni
here – a very fat siren. There has been some capital acting of
comedies by friends of Monsieur d'Albert – one of them is superior
to any actor of comedy I have ever seen . . . a handsome man of
fifty, full of wit and talent, and he married about a year ago.'
In another letter to the Brays, dated 15 February, she writes:

You know that George Sand writes for the theatre? Her
François le Champi – une Comédie, is simplicity and purity
itself. . . . We are going to have more acting here on Wednesday. Monsieur Chanel's talent makes Maman's *soirées* quite
brilliant. You will be amused to hear that I am sitting for my
portrait – at Monsieur d'Albert's request, not mine.

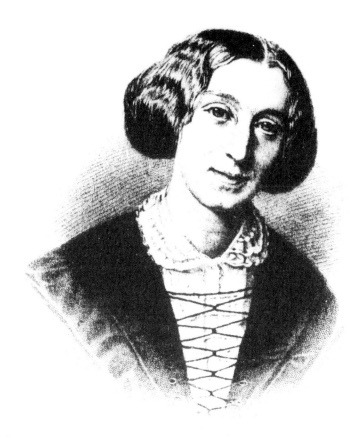

Miss Evans (George
Eliot) at thirty, by
Monsieur d'Albert

George Eliot left Geneva at the end of March, accompanied by
the devoted Monsieur d'Albert. Although departure had been
delayed in the hope of more spring-like travelling conditions, they
were obliged to cross the Juras on sledges, and evidently suffered
greatly from the extreme cold. Although it cannot be said that it
was a creative moment in her life, the Geneva interlude was
superbly therapeutic, and, to quote Mr Cross once again: 'It was
a peacefully happy episode . . . one she was always fond of
recurring to, in our talk, up to the end of her life.'

Notes

1. From the private diary of Francis Gye – possessed today by his family.
2. Byron himself claimed that Aeschylus's *Prometheus Vinctus*, which he had read as a boy, had partly inspired the poem.
3. *Manfred*. Scene 1.
4. *Praeterita,* John Ruskin.
5. *Praeterita*: Kenneth Clark, in introduction to the Oxford University Press edition, 1949.
6. *Praeterita*, John Ruskin.

CHAPTER *6*

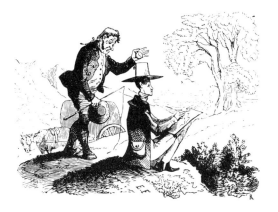

VISITING ARTISTS IN
GENEVA AND CHAMONIX

In the field of painting, a constant trickle of English artists had passed through Geneva and Chamonix during the second half of the eighteenth and early part of the nineteenth century. To a large extent these were young men, often travelling with their patrons, and usually on their way to Rome. The sheer magnificence of mountain, lake and waterfall – so different from the quiet, undulating landscape left behind, stimulated their senses; and they sketched and painted at every opportunity. Chamonix and its glaciers in particular exercised its fascination, just as it did on Ruskin and so many others. William Pars, Francis Towne, and J.R. Cozens belong to this group.

William Pars (1742–82) first travelled on the Continent in 1764, when he went with Richard Chandler and Nicholas Revett to Asia Minor, on a commission for the Dilettanti Society. Between his return and 1771, he accompanied Henry Temple, 2nd Viscount Palmerston, to the Continent, making drawings in Switzerland, the Tyrol and Rome.[1] 'The party travelled through Switzerland and the Tyrol and down through Italy. The water-colours which Pars produced anticipate the Swiss landscapes of Francis Towne and John Robert Cozens.'[2]

In 1774 Pars was awarded a further grant by the Dilettanti Society to continue his studies in Rome. He died aged barely forty, from a chill caught while standing and drawing in water at the Tivoli.

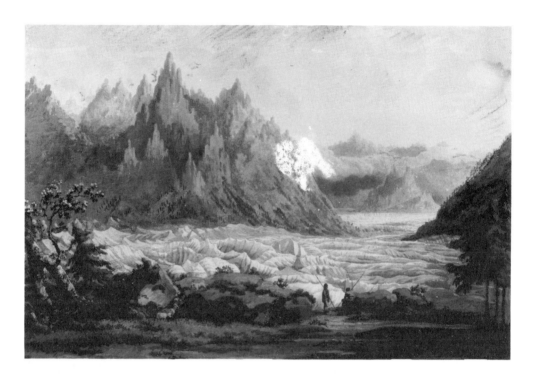

La Mer de Glace, Chamonix by William Pars (*Courtauld Institute of Art, London*)

Francis Towne (1740–1816) was born in Devon – probably in Exeter. At the age of thirty-two, he was made a member of the Society of Arts, and first exhibited at the Royal Academy three years later.

Towne's patrons were many, in particular the sixth Lord Clifford of Chudleigh, whose house Robert Adam had just built. After a tour of Wales, during which he perfected the tinted drawing and brought back some excellent work (including *The Salmon Leap, from Pont Aberglaslyn*), his thoughts turned towards the Grand Tour. Many of his fellow artists had been to Italy and Switzerland to paint. John Robert Cozens had only recently returned, and Towne may well have seen his work.

He began his tour in 1779, and seems to have gone by the direct route to Geneva – judging by the sequence of drawings – *Bridge over the Rhône at Geneva, The River issuing from the Lake* and *View of Geneva near the Confluence of the Arve and Rhône*.

In Rome he painted and drew with dedicated industry, producing exquisite work. Although Rome teemed with English artists at the time – notably Joshua Reynolds, Richard Wilson, Pars, Cozens, Humphry and Thomas Jones – Towne appears to

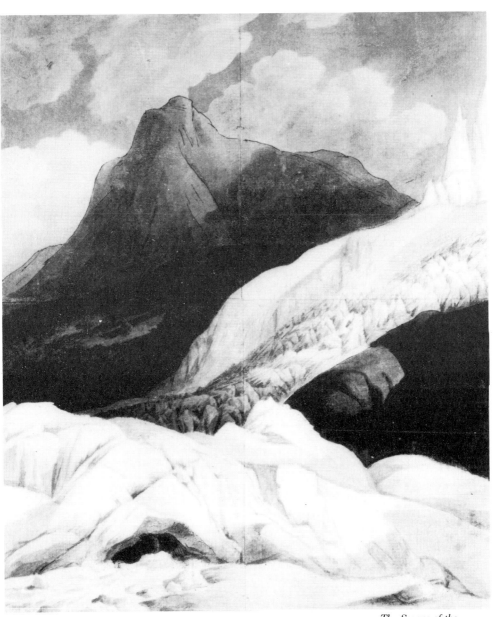

*The Source of the
Aveyron*, second
version, by Francis
Towne, 1781 (*The
Victoria and Albert
Museum, London*)

have kept very much to himself. While there, he met John 'Warwick' Smith, and they joined forces on the return journey, crossing into Switzerland by the Splugen Pass, and painting together a host of small water-colours. By September 1781, Towne was in Geneva again; and executed an aquarelle of *Lac Léman* which, as a composition, is particularly successful. He then took the road to Chamonix, and during the course of this expedition painted the remarkable water-colour *The Source of the Aveyron*.

'The impact of these immensities of nature on his somewhat timorous character fascinated him,' wrote Towne's biographer, A. Bury. 'Looking at them with the eye of the mind, Towne became, as it were, a medium, or *numéro* . . . Like all works of real poetic quality, *The Source of the Aveyron* pictures are mysterious both in spirit and deliverance. They are unique because he never improved on them.'[3]

He painted the same scene again, from a different angle.[4] The result, however, is much more stylised and less effective. A sketch, the *Mer de Glace*, followed, completed in 1793.

John Robert Cozens was the first of the really creative English water-colourists, and indeed used water-colours almost exclusively. His father, Alexander Cozens, was reputed to have been the natural son of Peter the Great and a Kent publisher's daughter. Unfortunately, there seems little foundation for this picturesque story, though John Robert's grandfather was principal shipbuilder to the Czar, and his father appears with certainty to have been born in Russia. Alexander was a landscape artist who worked almost exclusively in black wash or ink, using a curious technique of 'ink blots' to achieve almost abstract impressions. For many years William Beckford was Alexander's patron, and between 1782 and 1783, he took his son John Robert, then twenty-four, on a visit to Switzerland and Italy. This was not the first time that John Robert had visited the Continent. From 1776 to 1779, Richard Payne Knight, the archaeologist and art-collector, had taken him on his travels, journeying to Geneva and Chamonix and other parts of Switzerland before going on to Rome. (It is to this period that the drawing *Geneva from the North-West* belongs.) Thomas Jones, in his *Memoirs*, describes John Robert in Rome at that time, referring frequently to him as 'little Cozens'.

On his journey with William Beckford in 1782–3, John Robert executed what many regard as the finest water-colours he ever achieved. In effect, his style changed – becoming more tense, increasingly dramatic, richer in colour. In fact, his compositions are nearly all of nature at her most grandiose. Man and beast are depicted as minute forms in his scenes, as if to emphasise their helplessness in the face of natural forces.

Cozens' end was tragic. After 1792 he lost his reason, becoming, as Sir George Beaumont described it, 'paralytic', and totally unable to work. He died in 1797, having left a legacy to fellow artists which was to influence his contemporaries and their successors to an extraordinary degree. Constable called him 'the greatest artist who had ever touched landscape', and on another occasion commented, 'Cozens was all poetry'.

It is frustrating that so little is known about either of the Cozens. In the case of Alexander, we do at least have Beckford's occasional descriptive mentions of him, but of John Robert, we have virtually nothing, apart from the glimpses of his continental travels which his drawings and sketch-books give us. According to Oppie, their biographer, there was an unusually close relationship between father and son. John Robert seems to have received all his instruction from his father, while eclipsing him, 'as he himself was eclipsed by the generation of artists whom he in his turn had initiated'.

It is known that Alexander himself was painting in Rome in 1746. Oppie tells us that he left a note in connection with fifty-three of his drawings of Rome and Italy in general, saying that 'these drawings, and many more were lost in Germany by their dropping from his saddle when he was riding from Rome to England in the year 1746, and that they were purchased in Florence in 1776 by his son John Cozens, who, on arriving in London in 1779, delivered them to his father'.

The torch of John Robert Cozens was handed on in conspicuous fashion, for as young men, Turner and Thomas Girtin spent much time copying his water-colours. Tragically, Girtin died in 1802, at the age of twenty-seven, and it was in that year that Turner was elected a member of the Royal Academy. He set off on his first journey abroad, going first to Switzerland, to which he was naturally drawn by Cozens' landscapes. Here, he sketched and painted prolifically in the mountains round Geneva, finding, it appears, little to attract him in Geneva itself, though he later developed a sketch of *The Lake from Chambésy*, with the Môle in the middle distance, flanked by Mont Blanc.

During the next twenty years Turner often stayed at the Yorkshire home of William Fawkes, who was both friend and patron to him. Fawkes was a collector of water-colours, and in

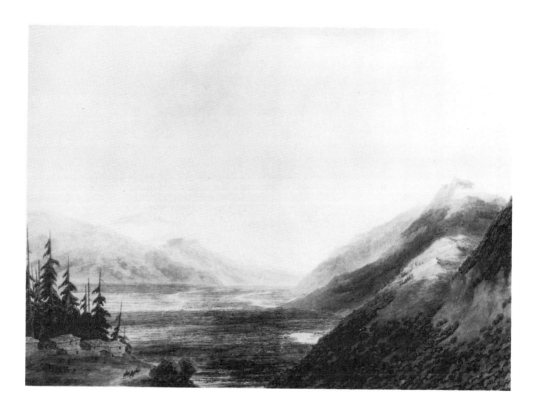

Le Pays de Valais, by
John Robert Cozens
(*Thomas Agnew & Sons
Ltd, London*)

1819 he held an exhibition at his London house. A press cutting
of the time gives the following account: 'On Tuesday Mr Fawkes
opened his house in Grosvenor Place for visitors . . . to see his
collection.' The writer goes on to describe the beauties of the
house '. . . without having previously known the owner's habits,
we should have pronounced it to be the house of an opulent and
manly-minded English landholder.' He conducts us mentally
through various rooms, including

'a suite of three handsome rooms, the last with a southern
aspect, and exhibiting the finest landscapes that we have ever
seen in water-colour. They are, we believe, all by Turner,
the Royal Academician, and almost all from the noblest
scenery in the world – the Swiss Alps; Views of Mont Blanc,
the Devil's Bridge, Chamouny, The Great St Bernard, the
Mer de Glace, mountains mingling with the clouds and rich
with all the effects of storm and sunshine, cataracts plunging
into an invisible depth, lakes shining like blue steel under the

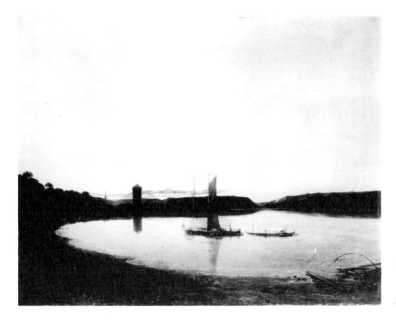

The Lake at Sunset, by
Francis Danby, 1839
(*Collection Musée d'art
et d'histoire, Geneva*)

Alpine sun, or clouded by forests hanging over them from
the hills, upland covered with vines and olives, and solitary
sweeps of splendid snow . . .'[5]

In the 1840s, when he was in his late sixties, Turner, who was
continually developing his style, returned to Switzerland, where he
painted a remarkable group of large water-colours. These myster-
iously beautiful works are considered to be some of the best achieve-
ments of his life, and his impressions of Geneva are masterly.

Another exceptionally gifted English artist – also connected
with Geneva and its surroundings – who appears never to have
received the recognition he deserved, and who throughout his life
was dogged by misfortune and frustration, was Francis Danby.
Danby, who with his family lived in Geneva between 1832 and
1836, is in many ways an enigma. Very little is known about him,
except through the accounts of his friends and contemporaries.
Recognition of his work has been further complicated by the fact
that his son, James Francis Danby, produced second-rate
imitations of Danby's later style and, in addition, he was much
copied by others.
Francis Danby was probably born in 1793, in Wexford,

Ireland. His father, James Danby, was an Irish country squire of moderate fortune, according to an article on Danby published in *The Art Journal* in 1855. When he was forty-one the Wexford Rebellion broke out. The loyalist James Danby narrowly escaped being murdered, and, in an atmosphere of continuing violence, he moved his family soon afterwards to Dublin.

In 1807, Francis' father died and his upbringing seems to have been dogged by poverty. He became an art student under the auspices of the Dublin Society, and made friends with two fellow students, George Petrie and James O'Connor, with whom he later went to London. From then on he considered himself an essentially English artist, and only rarely returned to his roots.

Over the next few years, Danby's style developed from the formally provincial into something more nearly approaching that of Turner. He settled in Bristol, and married secretly a 'very pretty-looking lass' shortly afterwards. This was in 1812, and Danby was only twenty. By 1818 he had four children, and his financial position was precarious. He kept things going by painting water-colours of local scenes and also gave drawing lessons.[6]

In 1820 he made his London debut with the *Upas Tree* which was shown at the British Institution. This, according to Danby's comments in the catalogue, was inspired by Erasmus Darwin's *The Love of the Plants*. Large, gloomy and horrific, the picture caused a considerable sensation. The following year Danby exhibited *Disappointed Love* at the Academy. In 1824, the artist Sir Thomas Lawrence himself purchased *Sunset at Sea*, and Danby moved to London. Cumberland, the art-expert, writing from Bristol to his son in London, commented, '. . . Danby is a good artist, but very opinionated, and is I fear a ruined man. He has a wife and children and pupils, but I believe through total thoughtlessness is over head and ears in debt; he has left this place hastily and secretly . . .'

Sunset at Sea was followed by *Enchanted Island*, which was highly acclaimed by the critics. In 1825 Danby exhibited *The Delivery of Israel out of Egypt* – 'astonishing the public, who scarcely expected such an exhibition of powers as were here displayed'. It was instantly bought by the Marquis of Stopford for five hundred guineas. At the end of that year, Danby was made an Associate of the Academy.

In 1826 he went to Norway, where he apparently found the romanticism of the landscape highly stimulating. But Norway was hardly the Alps, and in this way Eric Adams, his biographer,

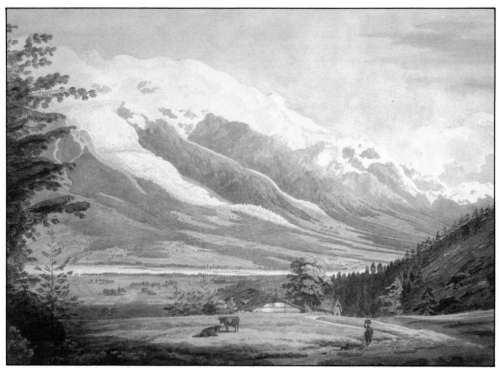

The Lower Part of the
Valley of Chamonix, by
William Pars (*British
Museum, London;
Photograph: Bridgeman
Art Library*)

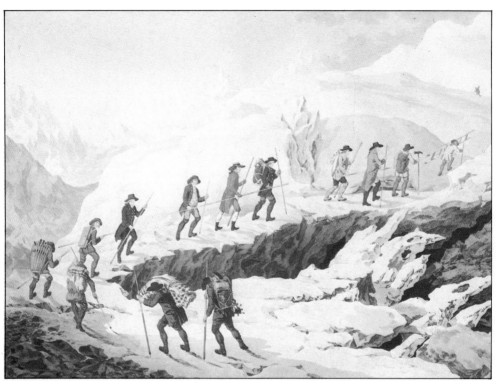

Monsieur de Saussure's
ascent to the summit of
Mont Blanc in August
1787, by Mechel
(*Photograph: Nicolas
Bouvier*)

suggests he was breaking new ground – both as traveller and artist.

For the Academy exhibition of 1826 he showed *Christ Walking on the Sea*. This was only tolerably well received, and neither it, nor *The Golden Age* which followed it, were sold.

This lean period continued until 1828, when Danby achieved his next success, *The Opening of the Sixth Seal*. This was enthusiastically received at the Academy, and William Beckford paid five hundred guineas for it. Colnaghi bought the engraving rights, and the British Institution gave him a prize. This raised a further five hundred guineas, and it looked probable that Danby would be appointed to the Academy to fill a recently vacated place. In the event, Constable beat him by one vote; and it seems clear that this was the result of some quarrel within the Academy, in which Constable may have been implicated.

Thereafter, Danby removed himself abroad – first to Paris and later to Geneva. The reasons are clouded in mystery, though it would seem that his unhappy marriage, together with difficult and souring relations with the Academy, were chiefly responsible. He returned briefly to complete *The Golden Age*, but quickly vanished again to Paris. As far as Eric Adams has been able to gather (helped by Hausermann's discoveries in the Geneva archives), he left his wife for a Welsh girl, Helen Evans, while Mrs Danby went off with his friend Poole. Danby removed his mistress and seven children to Paris, thereby indicating that his wife had first deserted all of them. He does not seem to have been creative while in Paris, and after a period of painting on the Rhine in 1813, he was forced to apply to the Academy for financial aid. They rose to the occasion, and the following year sent £50 to him in Geneva, where he was now living.

Danby arrived in Geneva in the summer of 1832. From the records of the Chambre des Etrangers (the organisation concerned with the surveillance of foreign visitors) it appears that he described himself, on arrival with 'wife' and children on 27 August, 1832, as 'Member of the Royal Academy', and that they initially stayed at the Hotel du Cheval Blanc. We know too that on 10 September, 1832 it is minuted: '. . . Danby, François, aged (?) [sic], native of England, holding a passport, accompanied by his wife, a son aged 16, and other children. He is staying at Les Paquis'.

A further minute informs us: 'On October 1st, 1832, Danby, described as *rentier*, deposited his passport and was given in exchange a *permis de séjour*'. (This was renewed, in all, thirteen times.) The following May the birth of a baby was registered in the *commune* of Cologny: 'Danby, Alfred, son of François Danby, aged 42, an Irish gentleman, and of Helen Evans, his wife, aged 27.' By this time the family were living at Montalègre, in a villa which was probably the one occupied by Shelley.

By November 1834 the minutes of the State archives reported the deteriorating financial affairs of 'François' Danby: '. . . [He] is running into debt and appears to have no means of subsistence'. The following week the committee registered increasing concern about him:

> . . . To be reconsidered when it expires, [they minuted:] the permit issued to the family of François Danby, Englishman, painter, of the Royal Academy, London, who has been reported as owing money to his baker, butcher, woodman, etc. He has ten children with him, of whom seven are by his wife, with whom he no longer lives, and three by a concubine with whom he cohabits. The oldest child is aged 18, and the youngest, 5 months. The two oldest intend to enter the service of His Britannic Majesty. Mr Danby admits to 100 louis of debts and has at present no means of paying them. He promises, however, to pay them before next May, when he intends to leave Geneva. He is strongly recommended by Monsieur le Pasteur Bouvier, who guarantees that the Danby household is so situated that the debts will be paid off as and when Monsieur Danby is paid for the pictures on which he is now at work.

The Minutes on 10 March 1835, read as follows: 'Danby [sic], François, Englishman, and his family, are still paying off their debts and now owe only some 50 louis. He is only staying on in the Canton in order to pay off his debts and intends to leave in the summer. The Committee decided to continue his permit for another six months.'

It appears from further research by Hausermann[8] that Danby sold four pictures at an exhibition at the Musée Rath on 2 August 1835. These were all bought by prominent Genevese of the time, though Hausermann was not able to trace them at the time he wrote his essay (1948). He did, however, discover a review of the exhibition in Le Fédéral of 18 September, 1835. After reviewing the exhibited work of other landscape artists (notably Calame, Guigon, Motu and Beaumont), the author wrote:

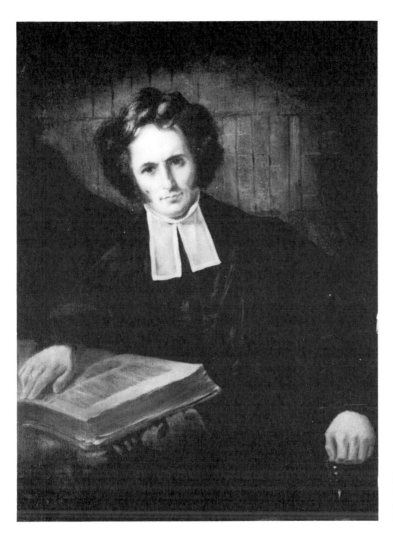

Pastor Bouvier
(*Bibliothèque Publique
et Universitaire,
Geneva*)

This section may be concluded with Monsieur Danby, the
Englishman who has become our guest. What can we say in
two words of this original painter, a poet to the very marrow
of his bones, whose works bear the print of an uncommon
genius? We could devote a whole article to the sunset on the
sea, which may be surprising, but is none the less true, and
even more than true; to the landscape gilded by a fiery sun,
which recalls the inspiration of Guaspre . . . and finally, the

Norwegian Lake, from which one cannot tear oneself away
. . . Suffice it to say that *Norwegian Lake* is the most
beautiful picture in the Salon; every artist will tell you the
same . . .

The results of the exhibition must have given the Chambre des
Etrangers relief and satisfaction. On 4 October 1835, it is
recorded in the minutes that Danby's *permis de séjour* had been
renewed: 'F. Danby (sic) who has now settled all his affairs; his
talent as a painter is appreciated and his pictures sell well.'

Soon afterwards the three eldest Danby sons left Geneva; and
on 18 April 1836, according to the records of the Chambre des
Etrangers, Danby himself reclaimed his passport, in order to take
his family to Paris.

As we have seen, Geneva boasted a lively intellectual life, and
there was a flourishing group of English residents there. Yet
somehow Danby does not seem to have made any real friends.
The one exception was Sir Samuel Brydges, an embittered old
Englishman with literary and aristocratic aspirations, whose
portrait Danby twice painted. Danby was clearly drawn to him,
and there is no doubt they had certain aspects of their lives in
common. At the same time, the Genevese undoubtedly
appreciated his work, and examples can be found in the private
collections of many of Geneva's old families, though there is no
evidence that Danby was on terms of personal friendship with any
of the buyers. Eric Adams points out, however, that Brydges
knew de Candolle; and there may have been a connection here, as
Mme. de Candolle was known to have possessed a small painting
of Danby's.[9] While Danby was in Geneva, Rodolphe Töpffer was
encouraging Swiss artists to take better advantage of the
magnificent scenery which surrounded them, though it is not
known whether his own works had a direct bearing on the
paintings of Calame or Diday, or how well the painters knew each
other.

Why was it that Danby removed himself from Geneva just
when considerable success had banished his finanacial burdens?
His friend, John Gibbons, writing to his son who was then in
Switzerland, quotes Danby as having told him that the Swiss
scenery left him unmoved, 'and that as a landscape artist he learnt
nothing'. Gibbons concludes that so much poverty and hardship
while he was in Geneva must have accounted for this attitude: 'As
Crabbe says, "it is the *mind* that sees", and his was not in the state
to see correctly.'

Danby spent the next two years in Paris. His work did not flourish, and he did much copying at the Louvre. By the spring of 1838 he wanted to leave. A mysterious illness killed off three, and perhaps four, of his children. It was a tragic time, and by the end of the year he was back in London, bringing with him *The Deluge*. This he exhibited in Piccadilly in 1840.

The Deluge has been considered Danby's most outstanding work, and Eric Adams comments: 'Perhaps Danby's personal distress added to the monumental gloom [of *The Deluge*]; for the manner seems to have particularly affected his work after his unhappy return to London.'

However, the picture re-made his reputation, and once again he established himself in London and began exhibiting at the Academy and the British Institution. Misfortune dogged him, though. He appears to have had further bad relations with the Academy, and three of his children left him and went to live with their mother. During this time, as had happened before, his friend John Gibbons was a tower of strength to him.

A few years later, Danby went to live in Exmouth, where he spent the last years of his life. *The Evening Gun*, exhibited at the Academy in 1848, was received with acclamation, and only reinforced his already high reputation with the public. He divided his time at Exmouth between painting and boat-building, which became an obsession with him. However, the death of John Gibbons, closely followed by that of his own son, Alfred (born in Geneva when the family first arrived there), shattered him.

Two of his pictures, *Calypso's Grotto* and *The Evening Gun*, were sent to the International Exhibition in Paris in 1855 to represent the English School of Painting. They were enthusiastically received – particularly *The Evening Gun*. The Academy's behaviour was deplored by art critics, who made no bones about the reason; and the Athenaeum commented: '. . . His [Danby's] absence from the Board of the Academy – on a ground far removed from artistic considerations – is the greatest reproach now lying against the forty [members] . . .'

He died at Christmas in 1860 an embittered man. His tomb is in the church of St John-in-the-Wilderness, Exmouth.

The difficulty with Francis Danby is that in spite of Hausermann and Eric Adams, he remains perversely shadowy as a character. While Maria Edgeworth's personality spills from every letter she writes (and how many there are!), we have almost nothing written by Danby, and such letters as exist are for the most part

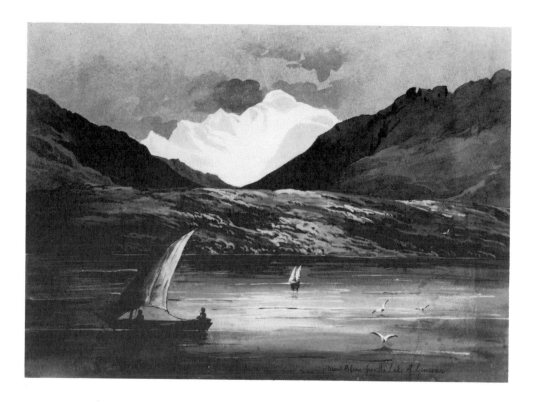

Mont Blanc seen from Geneva, by Edward Backhouse, *c.* 1830 (*Cabinet des Dessins, Collection Musée d'art et d'histoire, Geneva*)

concerned with the placement of his paintings and his difficulties in making ends meet. However, in an article in the *Cornhill Magazine* No. 968, Autumn 1946 Geoffrey Grigson comments, '. . . In one letter he [Danby] wrote: "Though the mind may be a diamond it will require a fresh setting if the body be as lead, and its very hardness and durability will help to destroy the setting" . . . Apart from this, one has no conception of Danby's thoughts, his philosophy.

Yet certain qualities seem to detach themselves from the admirable research done by Hausermann and Adams. Although unquestionably a muddler in all his personal affairs, Danby was a man who was loved and admired by his friends; a man with his own conception of honour; devoted and responsible where his children were concerned; leaping to the defence of the underdog; a man, in short, who did the best he could, in the face of much cruelty meted out to him. Surely it is of significance that the Chambre des Etrangers in Geneva – hardly a charitable organisation – should have treated him with almost tender solicitude! There must have been something unusually likeable about Danby.

Brief mention must also be made of those English travellers who as a matter of course recorded their impressions of the local scene in bulging sketch-books. These drawings and water-colours are inevitably of varying quality, though it is astonishing to discover the high standard often achieved. An impressive example of such amateurs is Edward Backhouse (1808-79).

Backhouse grew up in Sunderland, where his family were involved in collieries. He himself took no part in mining affairs. A cultivated man, with dilettante tastes, he was a good amateur painter and a student of natural history. He loved to travel and, judging by a collection of his work recently acquired by the Musée d'art et d'histoire in Geneva, must have toured Switzerland fairly extensively. At home he was a philanthropist, who showed great generosity to a number of charities. This versatile, gifted man was also an energetic liberal, and a devout Quaker. In 1854 he became a minister, and was the author of *Early Church History*.

Notes

1. Five of Pars' Swiss drawings, including the *Mer de Glace*, were later engraved by Woollett.
2. *British Watercolours, A Golden Age*, J.B. Speed Art Museum, Kentucky: Introduction and catalogue by Stephen Somerville.
3. *Francis Towne*, Adrian Bury, Charles Skilton Ltd, London, 1962.
4. In the Dyce Collection at the Victoria and Albert Museum.
5. *British Watercolours, A Golden Age*, J.B. Speed Art Museum, Kentucky. Introduction and catalogue by Stephen Somerville.
6. *Francis Danby: 'Varieties of British Poetic Landscape'*: Eric Adams, Yale University Press, 1973.
7. Hausermann: *The Genevese Background*.
8. Ibid.
9. This still remains in the de Candolle family.

CHAPTER 7

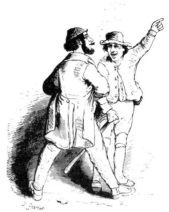

THE GLACIERS OF SAVOY

AND THE SALÈVE

There is no doubt whatever that the Alps exercised an irresistible fascination on English travellers, drawn to them in different ways as they were according to their own particular character. Geneva has its own skyline – the Mont Blanc range prowling in the background, its summit occasionally and gloriously above the clouds; the conical Môle in the near-distance; and, flanking the little canton, sometimes almost tangibly, Geneva's small mountain, the Salève. As we shall see, William Beckford cherished feelings about the Salève which were as romantic as they were dramatic. John Moore, on the other hand, gives a typically easy account, in another letter contained in *View of Society and Manners in France, Switzerland, and Germany*, of a visit he and the young Duke of Hamilton paid to the Mont Blanc range:

'That rare specimen, a perched tourist, swallowing chapter after chapter'; drawing by Rodolphe Töpffer (from *Nouveaux Voyages en Zigzag*)

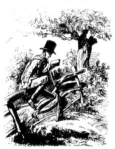

> . . . I returned a few days since from a journey to the Glaciers of Savoy . . . The wonderful accounts I had heard of the Glaciers had excited my curiosity a good deal, while the air of superiority assumed by some who had made this boasted tour, piqued my pride still more. One could hardly mention anything curious or singular without being told by some of those travellers, with an air of cool contempt – Dear Sir, – that is pretty well; but, take my word for it, it is nothing to the Glaciers of Savoy.
>
> I determined at last not to take their word for it, and I

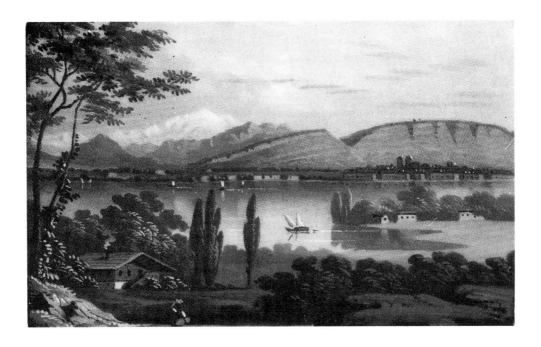

found some gentlemen of the same way of thinking. The party consisted of the Duke of H . . ., Mr U . . ., Mr G . . ., Mr K . . . and myself. We left Geneva early in the morning of the 3rd of August, and breakfasted at Bonneville, a small town in the duchy of Savoy . . .

View of Geneva and the Lake from Pregny, by Fanny Lang, *c.* 1850 (*Collection Musée d'art et d'histoire, Geneva*)

The party then proceeded to Cluse, and from there to Sallanches, where they stayed the night. Next morning they hired mules, and continued their journey towards Chamonix. In one village they saw peasants pouring into a church. Moore gives an almost childish (and very Protestant) account of the occasion. 'It was some saint's day – the poor people must have half-ruined themselves by purchasing gold-leaf, – Everything was gilded . . .' And he described the virgin in gold-papered gown holding in her arms an equally gilded infant with a 'periwig on his head, which was milk-white, and had certainly been fresh powdered'. He was further astonished to find, on the ceiling, 'a portrait of God the Father, sitting on a cloud, and dressed like a Pope, with the tiara on his head.'

They arrived at Chamonix about six in the evening, and next

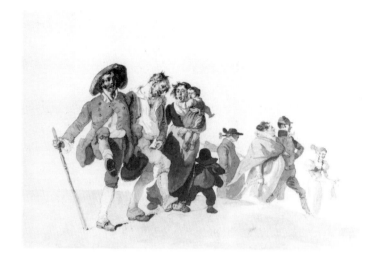

Group of peasants,
caricature by A. W.
Töpffer (*MAH,
Geneva; Cabinet des
Dessins*)

day 'began pretty early in the morning to ascend Montanvert,
from the top of which, there is easy access to the Glacier of that
name, and to the valley of ice.'

There follows an account of the young duke, who became
suddenly impelled to ascend the Aiguille du Dru. He was
followed by Mr G . . . . Neither, however, succeeded in reaching
their goal – neither having stopped to work out the best route. In
the end, the whole party had an agreeable picnic, and thereafter
proceeded to the Valley of Ice.

In 1777, at the age of seventeen, William Beckford (1760–1844)
arrived in Geneva to complete his education, accompanied by his
tutor the Reverend John Lettice. This first visit lasted more than
a year, and he fell romantically in love with the Salève. He
frequently returned in the years that followed, and on one
occasion, in 1786 (the year before Mont Blanc was conquered)
wrote:

> . . . I had long wished to revisit the holt of trees so
> conspicuous on the summit of Salève, and set off this
> morning to accomplish that purpose. Brandoin, an artist,
> once the delight of our travelling lords and ladies,
> accompanied me.

(On a previous occasion his travelling companion had been
J.R. Cozens the water-colourist – son of Alexander Cozens.)
Beckford describes how they reached the village of Moneti, and,

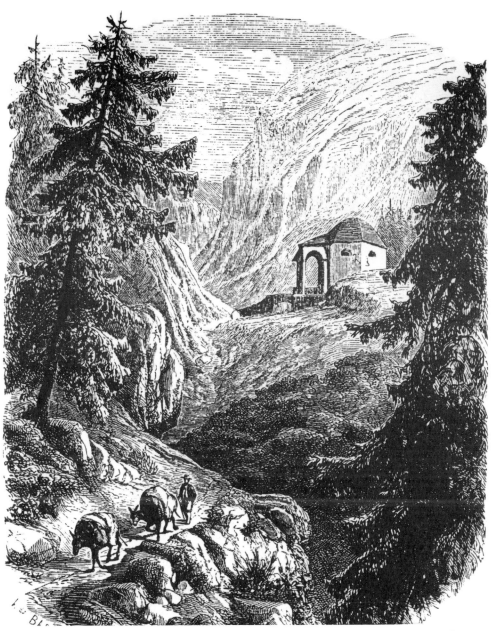

Mountain view by
Rodolphe Töpffer
(from *Nouveaux
Voyages en Zigzag*)

settling down in the shade of gigantic lime trees, dined 'as comfortably as a whole posse of withered hags, who seemed to have just alighted from their broom-sticks, would allow us'.

In due course, a sledge drawn by four oxen was prepared, to 'drag us up to the holt of trees'. Beckford then describes their gradual ascent on the straw-covered top of the sledge, with each bend of the track revealing to them new and vast views of the surrounding mountains. The evening was evidently overcast, and the susceptible Beckford's mood accorded with it, as he was overcome by mournful memories of his young wife Margaret, in whose company he had first visited this spot, and whose death a few months earlier had shattered him. What was more:

> We passed several chalets, formed of mud and stone, instead of the neat timber with which those on the Swiss mountains are constructed. Meagre peasants, whose sallow countenances looked quite of a piece with the sandy hue of their habitations, kept staring at us from crevices and hollow places.
>
> Gloomy feelings were partly dispelled when we reached the bold verdant slopes of delicate short herbage which crown the crags of the mountain. We now moved smoothly along the turf, brushing it with our hands to extract its romantic fragrance.
>
> Seating ourselves on the very edge of a rock cornice, we surveyed the busy crowded territory of Geneva, the vast reach of the lake, its coast, thickset with cattles, towns, and villages, and the long line of the Jura protecting these richly cultivated possessions. Turning round, we traced the course of the Arve up to its awful sanctuary, the Alps of Savoy, above which rose the Mont Blanc in deadly paleness, backed by a gloomy sky.

Before beginning the descent in pelting rain, Beckford was irritated at meeting some 'disappointed butterfly catchers, probably of the watch-making tribe'. This led him to make the following comment:

> . . . Silversmiths and toymen, possessed by the spirit of de Luc and de Saussure's lucubrations, throw away the light implements of their trade and sally forth with hammer and pickaxe to pound pebbles and knock at the door of every mountain for information. Instead of furbishing up

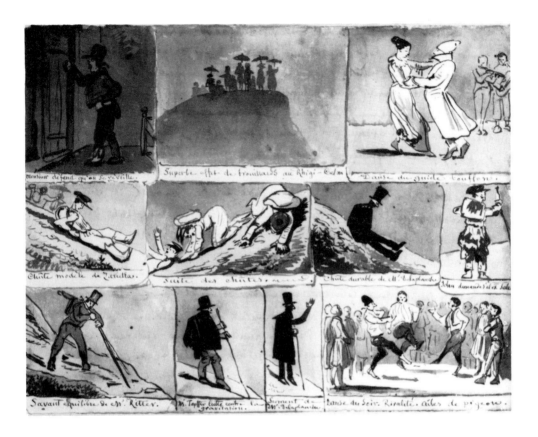

teaspoons and sorting watch-chains, they talk of nothing but quartz and feldspar . . . Squabbles arise about the genus of a coralite, or concerning that element which has borne the greatest part in the convulsion of nature . . . I cannot help thinking so diffused a taste for fossils and petrifactions of no very particular benefit to the artisans of Geneva, and that watches would go as well, though their makers were less enlightened.

Picturesque Journey, by Rodolphe Töpffer, 1829 (Cabinet des Dessins, Collection Musée d'art et d'histoire, Geneva)

Beckford, of course, was an odd character: product of a background compounded of immense wealth (Byron rightly called him son of the richest family in England); all-powerful connections; a lonely childhood spent in the hands of tutors – largely at Fonthill, the family home; and adulation of the kind only accorded to infant prodigies. A strange, Gothic figure, he produced his first book, *Biographical Memoirs of Extraordinary*

Painters, at the age of nineteen. This was later followed by his 'oriental' novel, *Vathek*, which made his name. It is claimed that much of the setting for *Vathek* was inspired by the wilder aspects of the Salève.

Early on, however, Beckford was involved in a scandal which marked his whole life. His biographer, Guy Chapman, believes he was intrinsically innocent in his relationship with the young William Courtenay;[1] but be that as it may, English society ostracised him for it. His more orthodox loves had been hardly orthodox, and in May 1783 his alarmed family eventually succeeded in marrying him off – at a still youthful age – to Lady Margaret Gordon. This marriage, after a sticky start, brought him much happiness. Margaret died shortly after producing their second daughter. They were by then living abroad to escape the scandal which pursued him, through which Margaret had unfailingly supported him. Beckford was devastated by her death, though the *mauvaises langues* claimed he had done away with her. The Swiss authorities at Vevey, where they were living, expressed their horror at the defamatory statements of the English news-rags, and actually signed a document to the effect that Beckford 'had always displayed towards his wife the utmost love and kindness'.[2]

Thereafter Beckford, leaving his two small girls with his mother after the funeral at Fonthill, fled back to Switzerland. He remained abroad until August 1793, when he returned to Fonthill, having commissioned James Wyatt to surround the estate with a great wall, within which was to be built a Gothic Abbey where, he announced, it was his intention to retire from the world. The building, when finished, was an unbelievable example of Gothic folly, and Chapman observes ironically that 'the palaces of battered Europe gave up their treasures' for the decoration of this hermitage.

A Genevese figure known to many young English students in the first half of the nineteenth century and much appreciated by his countrymen was Rodolphe Töpffer.

Rodolphe was born in Geneva in 1799, the son of A. W. Töpffer, himself a successful painter. As he grew up, his talent as an artist was to a large extent moulded by his passion for Hogarth, Rowlandson and Cruikshank, whom he called 'the great moralists: poets of the English School'.

At the age of twenty-five Töpffer created his own *pensionnat* where, over the years, he and his wife received a host of young foreigners many of whom, if not most, were English. At the same

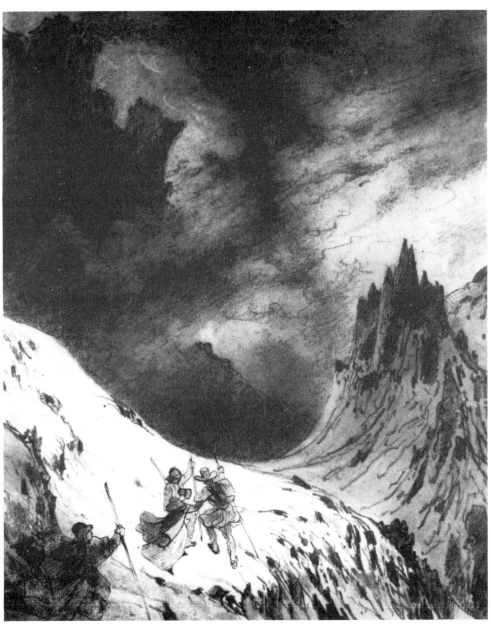

The Col d'Anterne, by
Rodolphe Töpffer
(*Cabinet des Dessins,
Collection Musée d'art
et d'histoire, Geneva*)

time, he pursued his career as gifted artist and commentator, publishing from time to time his *Voyages en Zigzag*, in which he immortalised the journeys he undertook with his students in the Alps. Töpffer had the keen eye of the cartoonist, and his comments – both in words and with his pen – are brilliantly perceptive.

He is, in short, extraordinarily amusing. In his *Nouvelles Genevoises*, he has a chapter on 'Le Col d'Anterne', a mountain-pass close to Chamonix. Töpffer describes his arrival at a tiny inn, where he hopes to both spend the night and pick up a guide. The only man available, he finds, is a chamois-hunter, and the only other guests at the inn, an English Milord and his daughter, have already engaged him. The story, which we are told is true, develops with splendid dialogue – the Englishman refusing to share the only guide, and generally behaving monstrously. (Töpffer renders his excruciating French phonetically.) In the event, Töpffer wakes early next morning to find father and daughter already gone. He decides to follow their footsteps in the snow. A snow-storm threatens. He catches them up at a moment when the storm engulfs them, and finishes by carrying the *jeune fille* down the mountain. Together with the guide, he brings them to safety, and has the satisfaction of Milord's gratitude. 'Vous ete mon ami, monsieur. Je n'ave pas d'autre chose que je pouve dire a vous!' ['You are my friend, sir. I have nothing more I can say to you!']

Notes

1. Son of Lord Powderham.
2. *The Travel-Diaries of William Beckford of Fonthill*; 2 vols, Guy Chapman, 1928.

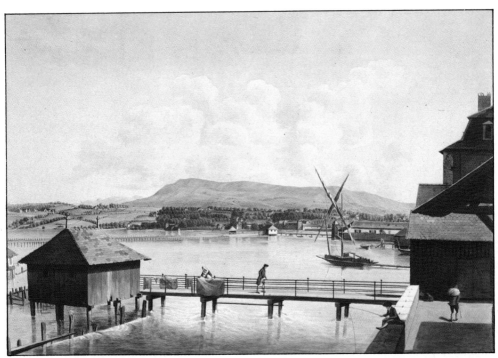

The Port des Barques
and the washerwomen
of the Coulouvrenière
in Geneva towards the
end of the eighteenth
century, by Ferrière
(*Photograph: Nicolas
Bouvier*)

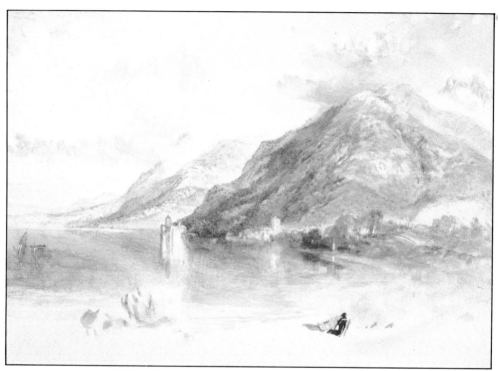

The Castle of Chillon,
Lake Geneva, from
Villeneuve, by
J. M. W. Turner (*The
Whitworth Art Gallery*)

CHAPTER 8

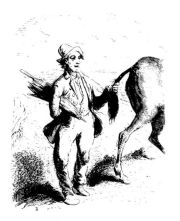

MONT BLANC

Mont Blanc, with the mystique attached to its serene, unworldly, and apparently impregnable summit, was unquestionably a focal point of attraction for visiting Englishmen – were they painters, poets, priests, or just healthy young men on the Grand Tour. As early as 1741, forty years before John Moore's dilettante expedition, William Wyndham, a young Englishman in his twenties from Felbrigg, Norfolk – together with a group of friends which included a certain Dr Pococke – set out to explore the 'Glaciers or Ice Alps, in Savoy'. C.E. Mathews tells us, in *The Annals of Mont Blanc*, published in 1895, that 'the valley in question was known to a few travellers, to Genevese bishops, and to local traders, but no account of it was ever given to the world'. Wyndham was part of 'quite a little colony of English' in Geneva at that time – mostly composed of young men like himself making a tour of Europe with their tutors. In the event, they not only saw 'the ends of the Glaciers which reach into the valley', but also succeeded in reaching the summit of 'the mountain', which was in fact the Montanvert. C.E. Mathews describes how:

the travellers all descended on to the ice, partly falling and partly sliding on their hands and knees . . . Having remained on the ice for half an hour, they drank like true Englishmen, to the health of Admiral Vernon and success to the British arms [the War of Jenkins' Ear]; and having regained the summit [the Montanvert] they descended to Chamonix – 'to the great astonishment of all the people of the place and even

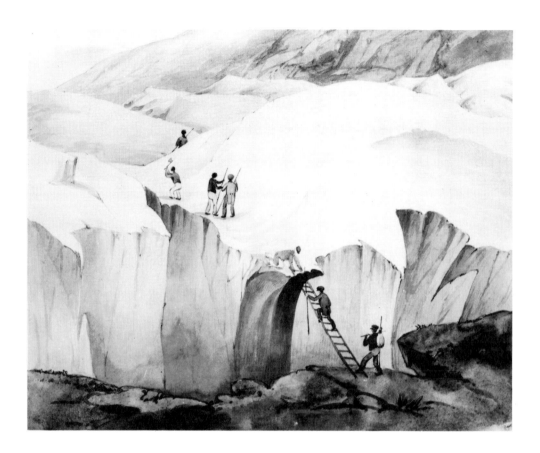

People scaling a glacier, by Edward Backhouse, c. 1830 (Cabinet des Dessins, Collection Musée d'art et d'histoire, Geneva)

of our guides, who owned to us they thought we should not have gone through with our undertaking'.

A few days later, the party arrived at Bonneville, and proceeded to climb the Môle.

Wyndham wrote a letter to Monsieur Arlaud – a well-known painter in Geneva – giving a full account of their journey to the Glaciers. After his departure from Geneva in August, 1742, the letter was widely circulated, and Pierre Martel, a Swiss engineer, decided to emulate his example. In his letter, Wyndham had stressed the need to take scientific instruments on such an expedition (having been ill-equipped himself in this respect), and this Martel and his party did. They succeeded in following the route taken by Wyndham and Pococke, and in due course returned to Geneva. Martel wrote a pamphlet on the journey, stating that he was an engineer and made thermometers. His pamphlet included Wyndham's letter 'to a friend' (i.e. Arlaud) and his own account, in the form of a letter to Wyndham. This pamphlet was in due course laid before the Royal Society, though it is curious to note that, far from taking the initiative in this respect, Wyndham himself made no official report, merely communicating a detailed account of his experiences to Arlaud. Wyndham and his friends were undoubtedly pioneers in high mountain climbing, and the *joie-de-vivre* with which their expedition was accomplished tells its own story. From then on Chamonix gradually began to be recognised as a centre for all attempts to climb Mont Blanc. Thus, mountaineering entered a new phase.

Meanwhile, that outstanding Genevese philosopher and scientist, Horace Benedict de Saussure (who, at the age of twenty-two, had become Professor of Philosophy at the Academy of Geneva) had conceived over the years a burning obsession with regard to Mont Blanc. In his *Voyages dans les Alpes*, he writes that from early childhood he had a passion for mountains, describing how in 1760 and 1761 he made it known in Chamonix' three parishes that he would handsomely reward anyone who could find a way to the summit of the 'Great White Mountain', indeed that he would even pay the time of those who were unsuccessful. It appears, however, that the men of Chamonix were by no means experienced mountaineers, and his offer was not immediately taken up.

In 1775 and 1783 there were two abortive attempts to climb the mountain, the three guides involved in the later effort reporting afterwards to de Saussure that they had been overcome by heat and sleep – one of them assuring him that were he (Jorasse) to try the same route again, he would carry only a parasol and a bottle of smelling-salts. This caused the Professor to observe drily:

> . . . When I picture to myself this big and robust mountaineer scaling the snows, holding a little parasol in one hand and a bottle of smelling-salts in the other, nothing gives me a better idea of the difficulty of this undertaking, and its absolute impossibility to people who have neither the heads nor the limbs of a good Chamouni guide.

A certain Monsieur Bourrit from Geneva – precentor at the cathedral and an artist who was a frequent visitor to Chamonix and believed he had been able to educate the men of the village in

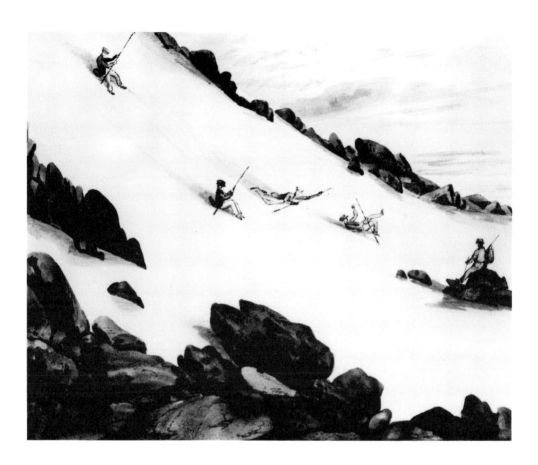

People sliding down frozen slopes, by Edward Backhouse *c.* 1830 (*Cabinet des Dessins, Collection Musée d'art et d'histoire, Geneva*)

the business of guiding – made several unsuccessful attempts to climb the mountain. In September 1785 he joined de Saussure in an expedition to reach the summit, de Saussure having had a small hut built on the mountainside, so that they could start from a higher level. Although the attempt was a failure, de Saussure, who took with him a variety of scientific instruments, was able to establish some interesting findings.

The following year, a young guide, Balmat, became separated from three other guides on the mountain, and, almost by accident, stumbled on a viable route to the top. Nightfall obliged him to desist, when he was within easy reach of the summit, and next morning he returned to Chamonix, where he confided his experiences to the village doctor, Dr Paccard. Dr Paccard was himself considering making an attempt on the summit, and Balmat offered to act as his guide.

Three weeks later they set out, and although the doctor frequently collapsed on the climb and, according to Balmat, had to be constantly forced on, they did in fact reach the summit by evening. Next morning, the doctor was snow-blind and was obliged to descend the mountain holding on to the strap of Balmat's pack.

Both men arrived back at Chamonix ravaged by sun and extreme cold. Balmat set out four days later for Geneva, only to find, when he reached de Saussure, that the news had already been conveyed to him by a shrewd Chamonix innkeeper hoping for a reward. De Saussure decided then and there to attempt the mountain himself, though for some strange reason he did not wish his decision to be known. However, weather conditions were such that it was a year before he was able to make the climb, and he eventually set forth on 1 August 1787. Jacques Balmat led a group of seventeen guides, and on 3 August they reached the summit. During the whole course of the expedition, de Saussure made constant notes with his meteorological instruments. The thinness of the air near the top made the going very hard, and he found he could not take more than fifteen or sixteen steps at a time without stopping to breathe.

> . . . I felt even from time to time a desire to swoon which obliged me to sit down . . . All my guides were in the same condition. We took two hours from the last rock to the top; and it was 11 o'clock when we got there.
>
> My first looks were directed to Chamouni, where I knew that my wife and her two sisters, with eyes fixed at the telescope, were watching my movements with uneasiness . . . I could then enjoy the grand spectacle which I had beneath my eyes . . . I could not believe my eyes, it seemed like a dream, to see beneath my feet these majestic peaks, these formidable Aiguilles, le Midi, l'Argentière le Géant, to get to whose very bases had been for me so difficult and so dangerous. I seized their bearings, their connection, their structures, and a single glance cleared away doubts which years of work had not been able to enlighten.[1]

Of this expedition, Edward Whymper wrote in 1896:

> Horace Benedict de Saussure was not a mountaineer, and did not pretend to be one; but his ascent of Mont Blanc gave an impetus to mountain exploration and, unwittingly, he

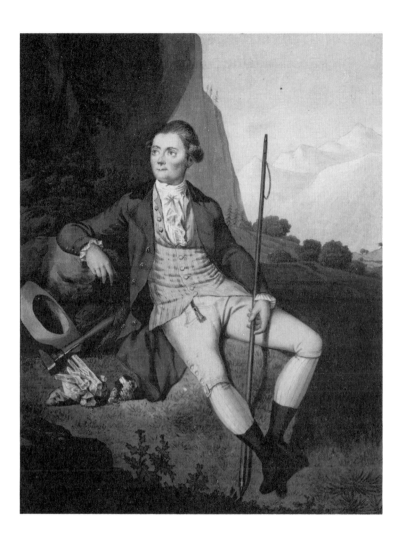

Horace-Benedict de
Saussure, engraving
after Juel, Geneva
(*Photograph: Nicolas
Bouvier*)

started the fashion for mountaineering. No sooner did he
return to Chamouni than a tourist who was there went off
and followed de Saussure's track. He was almost the first of
the mountaineering race. The Genevese philosopher
ascended the mountain to make physical, meteorological,
and geological observations; *Colonel Beaufoy* went up
principally to amuse himself. De Saussure does not,
however, seem to have done much in the way of attracting
others to Mont Blanc, for very few ascents were made in the
twenty-five years following 1787.[2]

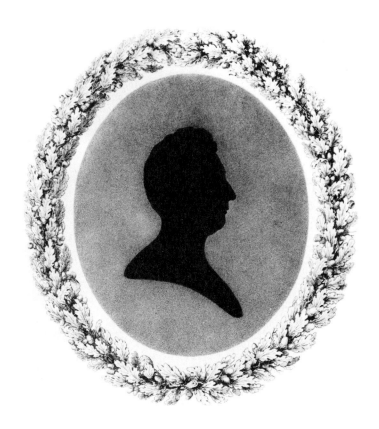

Silhouette of Colonel
Mark Beaufoy, from an
engraving by Henry
Brett (*Alpine Club
Collection, London*)

Whether or not Whymper was right in his estimate of Colonel
Beaufoy as being the 'first tourist' is open to judgement. In the
archives of the Alpine Club in London there are two documents
which give an unusually clear picture of Beaufoy's feat: the one, a
paper on the subject which he read to the Royal Society on 13
December, 1787; the other, written fifty years later, the original
of a letter from his son, Mark, to Mark's sister, in an elegant,
spidery, much-criss-crossed hand. 'Young' Mark went on a
'pilgrimage' to Chamonix in 1837, his principal object being to
seek out Cachat, his father's guide, at this time 'a very old man
but possessing all his faculties'.

. . . I was anxious to gain from him as much information
about the dear Pip [the family name for their father] as his
memory would allow, without giving him cause to suspect I
had any personal interest relative to the ascent made by the

first Englishman, for in the vale of Chamouni the inhabitants live by pleasing strangers and administering to their curiosity, so that inventions of all sorts of wonders would have been narrated to me had I announced myself Colonel Beaufoy's son.

Presumably Cachat imagined him to be a countryman of his father's, anxious to hear a first-hand account of the first conquest of Mont Blanc by an Englishman. It is of considerable interest to compare these two accounts, which corroborate each other in nearly all details. In that given by Michel Cachat (the substance of which is related by 'Young' Mark) there is a charming picture of Beaufoy's arrival.

> . . . At length, on August 3rd, 1787, Monsieur de Saussure reached the summit with 18 guides, carrying with him tent, bedding and many mathematical instruments with which he measured the height of the peaks by means of triangles.
>
> His ascent occupied four days as he occupied much time in measuring heights and other experiments. Scarcely had he quitted Chamouni when an English gentleman named Beaufoy, his wife, a nurse maid and infant daughter arrived and as usual with the guides, Cachat and others waited on the Colonel at the Inn who engaged them to conduct his Lady and self to Montanvert the next day.
>
> On descending the rough and difficult mountain to the source of the Aveyron which must have been a most fatiguing trial to our mother as in those days no footpaths existed, Cachat was surprised by the lady who was leaning on his arm telling him, 'My husband has a strong inclination to ascend Mont Blanc and I would wish you to spare neither money nor precautions in order that the excursion may be accomplished safely and successfully.'

Beaufoy's paper on the subject which he gave to the Royal Society reads as follows:[3]

> The desire of ascending to the highest part of remarkably elevated land, is so natural to every man; and the hope of repeating various experiments in the upper regions of the air, is so inviting to those who wish well to the interest of Science, that being lately in Switzerland, I could not resist the inclination which I felt to reach the summit of Mont Blanc.

One of the motives, however, which prompted the attempt, was much weakened by the consideration, that I did not possess, and in that Country could not obtain, the Instruments that were requisite for many of the experiments which I was anxious to make: and the ardour of common curiosity was diminished when I learned that Dr Paccard and his guide, who, in the year 1786 had reached the supposed inaccessible Summit of the hill, were not the only persons who succeeded in the attempt; for that five days before my arrival at the foot of the mountain, M. de Saussure, Professor in the University of Geneva, had gained the top of the Ascent.

But while I was informed of the Success which had attended the efforts of M. de Saussure, I was told of the difficulties and dangers that accompanied the undertaking; and was often assured with much laborious discussion that to all the usual obstacles, the lateness of the Season would add the perils of those stupendous masses of snow which are often dislodged from the steeps of the Mountain; together with the hazards of those frightful Chasms which present immeasurable Gulfs to the steps of the Traveller, and the width of which was hourly increasing . . .

Having formed my resolution, I sent to the different Cottages of the Vale of Chamouni . . . to enquire if any of them were willing to go with me as my assistants and my Guides; and had soon the satisfaction to find that ten were ready to accept the proposal. I engaged them all, and having announced to them my intention of setting out the next Morning, I divided among them provisions for three days, together with a Kettle, a Chafing Dish, a quantity of Charcoal, a pair of Bellows, a couple of Blankets, a long Rope, a Hatchet and a Ladder, which formed the stores that were requisite for the Journey.

After a night of much solicitude lest the Summit of Mont Blanc should be covered with clouds . . . I rose at five in the Morning and saw with great satisfaction that the mountain was free from vapour, and that the sky was everywhere Serene.

My Dress was a white flannel jacket without any shirt beneath, and white linen Trousers without Drawers. The Dress was white, that the Sun Beams might be thrown off; and it was loose that the limbs might be unconfined. Besides a Pole for walking, I carried with me Cramp Irons for the

heels of my Shoes, by means of which the hold of the frozen
Snow is firm, and in steep Ascents the poise of the body is
preserved.

My Guides being at length assembled, each with his
allotted burden; and one of them a fellow of great bodily
strength and great vigour of mind, Michael Cachat by name,
(who had accompanied M. de Saussure) having desired to
take the lead, we ranged ourselves in a line; and at 7 o'clock,
in the midst of the Wives and Children and Friends of my
Companions, and indeed of the whole Village of Chamouni,
we began our March.

The Colonel then describes the five-hour climb which led them
first to the Glacière de Bossons, and later to the Glacière de la
Côte, where they sat down beside a stream for a quick meal.

. . . Our Dinner being finished, we fixed our Cramp Irons to
our Shoes, and began to cross the Glacier; but we had not
proceeded far when we discovered that the frozen snow,
which lay in the Ridges between the waves of Ice, often
concealed, with a covering of uncertain strength, the
fathomless Chasms, which traverse this solid Sea; yet the
danger was soon, in a great degree, removed by the
expedient of tying ourselves together with the long Rope,
which being fastened, at proper distances, to our Waists,
secured from the principal hazard, such as might fall within
the openings of the Gulfs. Trusting to the same precaution
we also crossed upon our ladder, without apprehension, such
of the Chasms as were exposed to view; and sometimes,
stopping in the middle of the ladder, looked down, in safety,
upon an Abyss, which baffled the reach of vision, and from
the bottom of which, the sound of the masses of Ice, that we
repeatedly let fall, in no instance ascended to the Ear. In
some places we were obliged to cut footsteps with our
Hatchets; yet, on the whole, the difficulties were far from
being great, for in two hours and a half we had passed the
Glacière.

We now, with more ease and much more expedition,
pursued our way, having only snow to cross; and in two
hours arrived at a Hut which had been erected in the year
1786, by the order, and at the expense of Monsieur de
Saussure. The Hut . . . was in a state of such compleat
decay, that on my return the next evening, I saw, scattered

on the snow, many Tons of its Fragments which had fallen in my absence.

Immediately on our arrival, which was about five in the afternoon, the Guides began to empty the Hut of its snow; and at seven we sat down to eat; but our stomachs had little relish for food, and felt a particular distaste for Wine and Spirits. Water, which we obtained by melting snow in our Kettle, was the only drink we could bear. Some of the Guides complained of a heavy disheartening sickness, and my Swiss Servant, who had accompanied me at his own request, was seized with excessive vomiting, and the pains of the severest Head Ache. But from these Complaints, which apparently arose from the extreme lightness of the Air in these elevated regions, I myself and some of the Guides were free, except, as before observed, that we had little appetite for food, and a strong aversion to the taste of spirituous Liquors. We now prepared for rest, on which two of the Guides, preferring the open Air, threw themselves down at the entrance of the Hut, and slept upon the Rock. I too was desirous of sleep . . . my repose was soon disturbed, by the noise of those masses of Snow which were loosened by the wind from the heights around me, and which, accumulating in bulk as they rolled, tumbled at length from the Precipices into the Vales below, and produced upon the Ear, the effect of redoubled bursts of Thunder.

At two o'clock I threw aside my Blankets, and went out of the Hut to observe the appearance of the heavens. The Stars shone with a lustre that far exceeded the brightness which they exhibit when seen from the usual level; and had so little tremor in their light, as to leave no doubt in my Mind, that if viewed from the summit of the Mountain they would have appeared as fixed points . . . At the time I rose, my Thermometer, which was on Fahrenheit's scale, and which I had hung on the side of the Rock without the Hut, was eight degrees below the freezing point. Impatient to proceed and having ordered a large quantity of snow to be melted, I filled a small Cask with water for my own use, and at three o'clock we left the Hut. Our Route was across the snow; but the Chasms which the Ice beneath had formed, tho' less numerous than those we had passed the preceeding day, embarrassed our ascent. One in particular had opened so much in the few days that intervened between M. de Saussure's expedition, and our own, as for a time, to bar the

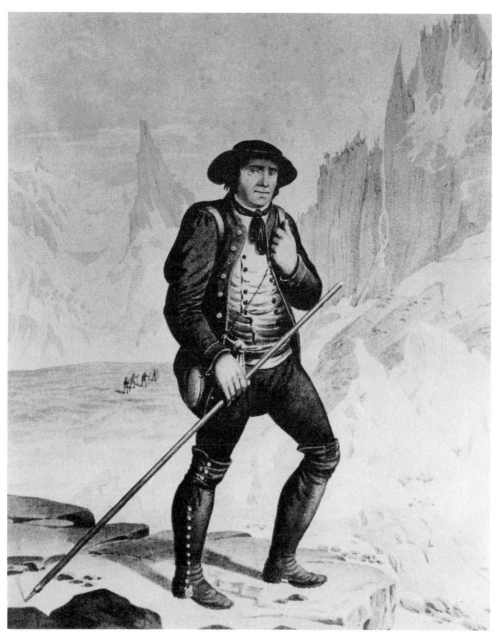

Jean-Michel Cachat,
known as 'the Giant'
(*Alpine Club Collection,
London*)

hope of any further progress; but at length, after having wandered with much anxiety along its bank, I found a place which I thought the ladder was sufficiently long to cross. The ladder was accordingly laid down and was seen to rest on the opposite ledge; but its bearing did not exceed an inch on either side. We now reflected, that if we should pass the Chasm, and its opening, which had enlarged in the least degree, no chance of return would remain. We further reflected, that if the Clouds, which so often envelop the hill, should rise, the hope of finding, amidst the thick fog, our way back to this only place in which the gulf, even in its present state was passable, would be little less than desperate. However, notwithstanding these alarming apprehensions, the Guides after a Moment's Pause consented to go with me and we crossed the Chasm. We had not proceeded far, when the thirst, which, since our arrival in the upper regions of the Air, had been always troublesome, became almost intolerable. No sooner had I drank than the Thirst returned, and in a few minutes my Throat became perfectly dry . . . The Guides were equally affected. Wine they would not taste; but the moment my back was turned, their mouths were eagerly applied to my Cask of Water. Yet we continued to proceed till 7 o'clock, when having passed the place where M. de Saussure who was provided with a tent had slept the second night, we sat down to Breakfast. At this time the Thermometer was four degrees below the freezing point.

We were now at the foot of Mont Blanc itself, for tho' it is usual to apply that term to the whole assemblage of several successive Mountains, yet the name properly belongs only to a small mountain of a Pyramidal Form, that rises from a narrow plain, which, at all times is covered with Snow. Here the thinness of the Atmosphere began to affect my head with a dull and heavy pain. I also found an acute sensation of Pain, very different from that of weariness, immediately above my Knees.

Having finished our repast, we pursued our Journey, and soon arrived at a Chasm which could not have existed many days; for it was not formed at the time of Monsieur de Saussure's descent.

Misled by this last Circumstance (for we concluded as he had seen no rents whatever from the time that he passed the place on which he slept the second night, none were likely to be formed) we had left our ladder about a League behind, but as the Chasm was far from being wide, we passed it on the Poles that we used for walking; an expedient which suggested to me that the length of our ladder might be easily increased by the addition of several poles laid parallel and fastened to its end; and that the hazard of finding our retreat cut off, from the enlargement of the Chasms, might by this means be materially diminished. At this place I had an opportunity of measuring the height of the Snow which had fallen in the preceding winter, and which was distinguished by its superior whiteness from that of the former year. I found it to be five feet. The Snow of each particular year appeared as a separate Stratum. That which was more than a twelvemonth old was perfect Ice, while that of the last Winter was fast approaching to a similar state.

At length, after a difficult ascent, which lay among Precipices, and during which we were often obliged to employ the Hatchet in making a footing for our feet, we reached and reposed ourselves on a narrow flat, which is the last of three from the foot of the small mountain, and which according to M. de Saussure, is but 150 Fathom below the level of the summit. Upon this Platform I found a beautiful dead Butterfly, the only appearance which, from the time that I entered on the Snow, I had seen of any animal.

The Pernicious effects of the thinness of the air were now evident on us all. A desire, almost irresistible, of Sleep came on. My Spirits had left me. Sometimes, indifferent as to the event, I wished to lie down: at others I blamed myself for the expedition, and tho' just at the Summit, had thoughts of returning back without accomplishing my purpose. Of my Guides, many were in a worse situation; for being exhausted by excessive vomiting, they seemed to have lost all strength both of mind and body. Shame at length came to our relief. I drank the last pint of water that was left, and found myself amazingly refreshed; yet the pain in my Knees had increased so much, that at the end of every 20 or 30 Paces I was obliged to rest till its Sharpness had abated. My lungs with difficulty performed their office; and my Heart was affected with violent Palpitations.

At last, however, but with a sort of Apathy which scarcely admitted the sense of Joy, we reached the summit of the mountain; when six of my Guides and with them my Servant, threw themselves on their Faces, and immediately

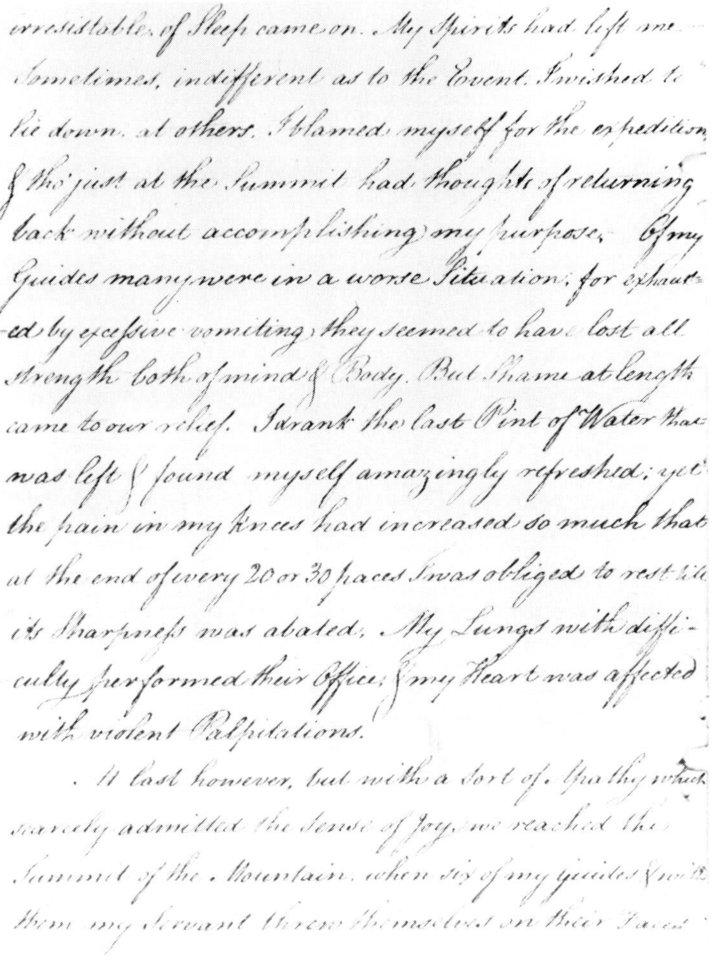
irresistable of Sleep came on. My Spirits had left me
Sometimes, indifferent as to the Event. I wished to
lie down at others. I blamed myself for the expedition
& tho' just at the Summit had thoughts of returning
back without accomplishing my purpose. Of my
Guides many were in a worse Situation; for exhaust-
-ed by excessive vomiting, they seemed to have lost all
strength both of mind & Body. But Shame at length
came to our relief. I drank the last Pint of Water that
was left & found myself amazingly refreshed; yet
the pain in my Knees had increased so much that
at the end of every 20 or 30 paces I was obliged to rest till
its Sharpness was abated. My Lungs with difficulty performed their Office; & my Heart was affected
with violent Palpitations.

At last however, but with a sort of Apathy which
scarcely admitted the Sense of Joy, we reached the
Summit of the Mountain, when six of my Guides & with
them my Servant threw themselves on their Faces

Facsimile of an extract from Colonel Beaufoy's account to the Royal Society of his ascent of Mont Blanc (*Alpine Club Collection, London*)

fell asleep. I envied them their repose but my anxiety to obtain a good observation for the Latitude subdued my wishes for Indulgence. The time of my arrival was half an hour after ten in the Morning; so that the hours which had elapsed from our departure from Chamouni were only 27 1/2; ten of which we had passed in the Hut. The summit of the Hill is formed of Snow, which spreads itself into a sort of Plain that is much wider from East to West than from North to South, and in its greatest width is perhaps thirty yards. The Snow is everywhere hard, and in many places is covered with a sheet of Ice.

When the Spectator begins to look around him from this elevated height, a confused impression of Immensity is the first effect upon the mind; but the blue colour, deep almost to blackness, of the Canopy above him soon arrests his attention. He next surveys the Mountains around him, many of which from the clearness of the Air, are to his Eye, within a Stone's throw from him, and even those of Lombardy . . . seem to approach his neighbourhood; while, on the other side, the vale of Chamouni, glittering with the Sun Beams, is to the view directly below his Feet, and affects his head with giddiness. On the other hand, all objects of which the distance is great and the level low are hid from his Eye by the blue vapour which intervenes, for I could not discern the Lake of Geneva . . .

As the time of the Sun's passing the Meridian now approached, I prepared to take my observation. I had with me an admirable Hadley's Sextant, and an artificial Horizon; and I corrected the refraction of the Sun's Rays by the Thermometer which I had brought with me, and by the descent of the Barometer as determined by M. de Saussure. Thus I was enabled to ascertain with Accuracy, the Latitude of the Summit of Mont Blanc, and found it to be 45° 50'.

I now proceeded to such other observations as the few Instruments which I had brought permitted me to make. At 12 o'clock the Mercury in the Thermometer stood at 38° in the Shade. At Chamouni at the same hour, it stood, when in the shade, at 78°.

I tried the effect of a burning Glass on Paper, and on a piece of Wood which I had brought with me for the purpose; and found (contrary, I believe, to the generally received opinion) that its strength was much greater than in the lower regions of the Air.

Having continued two hours on the Summit of the Mountain, I began my descent at half an hour after 12. I found that, short as my absence had been, many new rents were opened, and several of those I had passed in my ascent, were become considerably wider. In less than six hours we arrived at the Hut in which we had slept the night before; . . . Our Evening's repast being finished, I was soon asleep; but in a few hours was awakened with a tormenting pain in my Face and Eyes. My Face was one continued Blister, and my Eyes I was unable to open; nor was I without apprehension of losing my sight for ever, till my Guides told

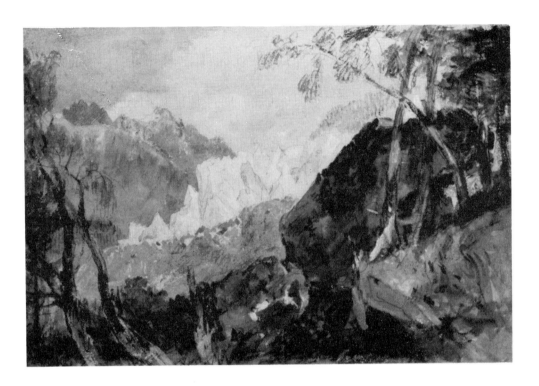

me that in a few days I should recover their use; and that if I had condescended to have taken their advice of wearing, as they did, a Mask of Black Crêpe, the accident would not have befallen me. After I had bathed my Eyes with warm water for half an hour, I found, to my great satisfaction, that I could open them a little; on which I determined upon an instant departure, that I might cross the Glacière de la Côte before the Sun was risen sufficiently high for its Beams to be strongly reflected from the Snow. But unluckily the Sun was already above the Horizon; so that the pain of opening my Eyes in the bright Sun shine, in order to avoid the Chasms and other hazards of my Way, rendered my return more Irksome than my Ascent. Fortunately one of the Guides, soon after I had passed the Glacière, picked up, in the Snow, a pair of green Spectacles, which M. Bourrit had lost, and which gave me wonderful relief. [Bourrit had made yet another unsustained attempt to climb the Mountain on the return from the summit of M. de Saussure. He had dropped his glasses, and had suffered much with his eyes as a result.]

Glacier de Bosson, by J. M. W. Turner (*Bacon Collection, Courtauld Institute of Art, London*)

At 11 o'clock on the 10th August, after the Absence of 52 hours, of which twenty were passed in the Hut, I returned again to the village of Chamouni.

From the want of Instruments, the observations I made were few – yet the effects which the Air, in the heights I visited, produces on the human body, may not perhaps be considered by the Society as altogether uninteresting; nor will the proof which I made of the power of the Lens on the summit of Mont Blanc, if confirmed by future experiments, be regarded as of no account in the Theories of Light and Heat. At any rate, the having determined the Latitude of Mont Blanc may assist the Astronomical Observations of such persons as shall visit it in future; and the knowledge which my Journey has afforded, in addition to that which is furnished by M. de Saussure's, may facilitate the ascent of those who, with proper Instruments, may wish to make, in that elevated level, experiments in Natural Philosophy; a business which if others, who are better qualified should not undertake, I shall myself at some future period, probably pursue.

The unfortunate Bourrit, who had remained on in Chamonix after de Saussure's departure to nurse his eyes, wrote as follows in a letter to Miss Craven, dated 13 August:

... Mes yeux depuis lors ont été enflammés, et ils l'étoient encore après le départ de M. de Saussure pour Génève, lorsque j'appris qu'un Anglois s'étoit annoncé ici pour monter le Mont Blanc; ma situation m'ota l'espoir de le suivre. C'étoit Monsieur de Beaufoix, Astronome et Physicien. Jeune, plain d'ardeur et de courage, il partit le mercredi 8 du courant avec 10 guides et son domestique: je le vis atteindre le sommet le jeudi, et vendredi il fut de retour le matin. Il a beaucoup souffert; il s'est cru aveugle et son visage a été boursoufflé ... Son épouse, qui n'a que 19 ans, a joui du succès de son epoux ... Sur l'insouciance que l'on éprouve au Mont Blanc, je demandai à M. Beaufoix, et en présence de son aimble épouse, si sur le Mont Blanc il avait pensé à elle? Il répondit par un *non* absolu ... [My eyes were inflamed from then onwards, and they remained so after the departure of Monsieur de Saussure for Geneva. When I learned that an Englishman had arrived here to climb Mont Blanc, my predicament removed all hope of my

following him. This was Monsieur de Beaufoix, the
Astronomer and Physician. Young, full of keenness and
courage, he left on Wednesday 8 [August] with ten guides
and his servant: I saw him reach the summit on Thursday,
and on Friday he arrived back in the morning. He suffered
greatly; he thought he was blind and his face was bloated.
His wife, who is only nineteen, was delighted with her
husband's success . . . Concerning the apathy that one feels
on Mont Blanc, I asked Monsieur Beaufoix, in the present of
his charming wife, if he had thought of her on Mont Blanc?
He replied with an emphatic '*no*'.]

Inevitably, curiosity is aroused by Colonel Mark Beaufoy.
What were his origins? And why did he suddenly appear on the
Chamonix scene, marching without fuss up the formidable
Mountain, and marching thereafter into history?
The Alpine Club hold in their archives a booklet entitled
Leaves from a Beech Tree, by Gwendolyn Beaufoy.[4] Gwendolyn
was a descendant of Mark Beaufoy by marriage, and while
turning out the attic of their house in Lambeth, in the late 1920s,
she came across a series of papers relating to her husband's
family. She pieced these together as well as she could, and in 1930
published them privately.
The Colonel's father, Thomas Ramell, was apprenticed to the
Distillery in Bristol in 1734, and 'was so impressed by Hogarth's
pictures of Gin Lane that he went over to Holland and there
learned the art of making vinegar, which has been the business of
the Beaufoy family ever since 1740.'
Mark was born in 1764. His mother died when he was only
eight, and he grew up in a strong Quaker atmosphere at the family
home in Cuper's Gardens, Lambeth. When only twenty he fell in
love with his first cousin Margaretta and, in the face of his father's
objections, eloped with her to Gretna Green. It is interesting to
note that Margaretta herself can only have been sixteen at the
time of the elopement. Almost at once they moved abroad, and
lived in Neuchatel for three years. Their first two children were
born there. Gwendolyn, in *Leaves from a Beech Tree*, writes:

Mark . . . was a brilliantly clever man, and besides writing
various articles on scientific matters, navigation and
astronomy, had the honour of being the first Englishman to
ascend Mont Blanc. He had an Astronomical Observatory at
Bushey Heath, and corresponded with the leading

astronomers of his day both at home and abroad. His wife was an excellent mathematician and assisted him greatly in his calculations.

Among his many contributions to science was the leading part he played in establishing in 1791 the Society for the Improvement of Naval Architecture, which in turn led to an important series of experiments carried out under his care. He was also a major contributor in the fields of hydraulic experiments, magnetic discoveries and astronomy, as well as being a Fellow of the Linnean Society. In 1817 he was admitted to the Royal Society.

After the celebrated climb, we learn from Gwendolyn Beaufoy that Mark and his family returned to England, living first in Great George Street, London, and then in Hackney Wick.[5]

Edward Whymper tells us more about the climbing conditions which existed on Mont Blanc, after 1787:[6]

> . . . in the twenty-five years after Mont Blanc was conquered there were only half-a-dozen other ascents, and the persons who went up had to be nursed and cared for like so many children. Even the professional guide went about in those days in a fashion which would now be thought absurd. The ice-axe was almost unknown, and when difficulties were met with they had to be avoided or circumvented.

Describing changes which were gradually made in the established routes, he tells us,

> . . . *Mr. Auldjo*, who went up Mont Blanc on August 9th, 1827, says he crossed the Grand Plateau towards the left, 'leaving the old route, which led right across the plain'; and later on, when above the *Rochers Rouges*, he mentions that he 'came again into the old line of ascent, which we had quitted on the Grand Plateau', and remarks that the new line was first taken by 'Messrs Hawes & Fellows, on the 25 July last, we having followed the route which these gentlemen had discovered'.

Auldjo thoughtfully left a bottle of brandy in the Hut at the Grands Mulets, for the next man to attempt the climb. Three years later, Edward Bootle Wilbraham came to Chamonix with a Captain Pride and the Comte de Hohenthal. The weather was

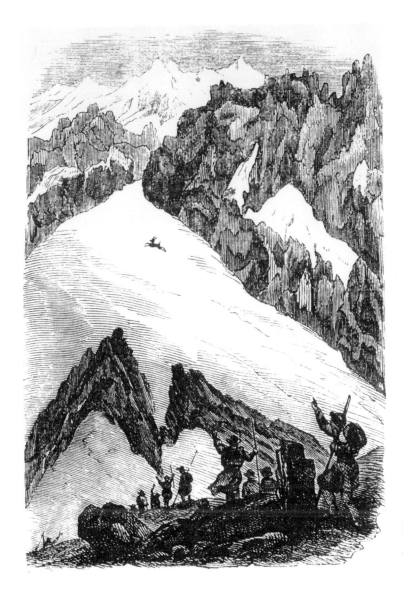

Drawing by Rodolphe
Töpffer (from
*Nouveaux Voyages en
Zigzag*)

fine and clear, and he was tempted to try the climb. He
approached the guide Couttet, and with great difficulty
persuaded him to prepare an expedition with six guides. They set
off on 2 August, and reached the Grands Mulets seven hours
later. They were enchanted to find Auldjo's brandy, and
Wilbraham instructed his guides to leave some bottles of wine for

whoever his successor might be. They slept under canvas, and at
2.30 a.m., were up and ready to go. Four hours later they arrived
at the Grand Plateau, where they stopped for breakfast. As they
passed the foot of the *ancien passage*, Couttet pointed to the
crevasse in which three of Dr Hamel's guides were engulfed,
saying: 'They are there!' (Dr Hamel left Chamonix with two
young Englishmen, Durford and Henderson, on 18 August 1820.
Near the *ancien passage* they were overwhelmed by an avalanche,
and were hurled into a crevasse, which was instantly covered by
thick snow. In 1861, the three victims were disgorged at the
Glacier de Bosson.) Wilbraham and his party duly reached the
summit, and like others before and after, they collapsed from
exhaustion. They soon recovered, however, and returned without
problems of any kind. In 'An Ascent of Mont Blanc in August
1830', published in the *Keepsake* in 1832, Wilbraham described
how he rode into Chamonix on a mule, to be lionised by all, 'the
visitors asking him the most absurd questions imaginable'.

Four years later, in mid-September 1834, Dr Martin Barry
(Doctor of Medicine of Edinburgh University, President of the
Royal Medical Society of Edinburgh and Fellow of the Royal
Society of that city), was on a walking tour in Switzerland. A view
of Mont Blanc from the Col de Balme had such an effect on him
that he decided then and there to make the climb. Despite the
warning of guides that the season was too advanced, with already
much snow, he succeeded in persuading six of them to accompany him. He at once set about preparing his expedition,
managing to borrow clothes at his hotel.

At 8.30 next morning, the party left for the ascent. Great
difficulty was experienced on the glacier, on account of the
lateness of the season combined with the end of an unusually hot
summer. Dr Barry had to be forcibly pulled up the rocks to the
Grands Mulets by the chief guide, Joseph Marie Couttet, who
presented him with a certificate saying that although he, Couttet,
had made the climb nine times, never had he had such difficulty
in reaching the rocks. They passed a good night, and Barry, who
must have been something of a romantic, was entranced by the
effect of brilliant moonlight on the mountain.

Next day they left at 5 a.m. – much delayed again by the soft
snow. By the time they reached the Mur de la Côte, the doctor
was at exhaustion-point. According to pattern, he was attacked by
a feeling of complete indifference, and somehow managed to
accomplish the final stage to the summit in a near-fainting
condition, having been actually walking nearly twenty hours.

Once there, he soon recovered, made some scientific experiments, and then proceeded to revel in the splendour of the scene. The return journey caused little problem, apart from occasional falls into hidden crevasses, from which Barry was apparently easily rescued.[7]

The following evening he gave a party for his guides. Old Jacques Balmat, then aged seventy-three, joined them, and further enlivened the occasion by relating his own experiences on the mountain, nearly half a century before.

H.M. Atkins, 'a very young gentleman' pursuing his studies in Geneva in the year 1837, paid a holiday visit to Chamonix in the month of August. Here he met another Englishman, Pidwel, and a Swedish officer of artillery, Hedrengen. The three determined to make the ascent together. They engaged Michel Balmat as chief guide, who, when he had accepted the engagement, begged permission to pass the day with his family. Atkins was greatly struck with this fact, which convinced him that he was engaged in a very perilous undertaking. The guides, he tells us, 'displayed no eagerness; there was a solemnity in their countenances and in the manner in which they laid their plans; they collected in little groups about the village and consulted in a low voice.'

A certain Countess K . . . who was at Chamonix at the time begged and prayed him not to undertake the expedition. An Irish gentleman, too, showed him great attention, read to him the history of the Count de Tilly who had his feet frozen, offered to make his will, and consoled him by the information that if he were lost and his body discovered after an interval of ten years, it would be easily identified. Nevertheless, the party, consisting of thirteen people, started at seven on the morning of the 22 August.

At eleven they reached the Pierre à l'échelle, the three travellers, if the pictures which Atkins subsequently published may be relied upon, wearing tall hats. Michel Balmat took a dog with him, the first which ever reached the mountain's summit. Atkins had never previously been upon a glacier, but Pidwel and Hedrengen had both climbed in Norway and were expert mountaineers. They all reached the sleeping place at the Grands Mulets at half-past four. The weather was beautiful, but Atkins was too much excited to sleep, and 'thought of home and all that was most dear to him'. They were awakened at 2 o'clock and:

at a quarter before seven they were on the *Grand Plateau* and partook of frozen fowls, frozen bread, and frozen wine. Atkins was well clothed, wearing lambs' wool stockings, two

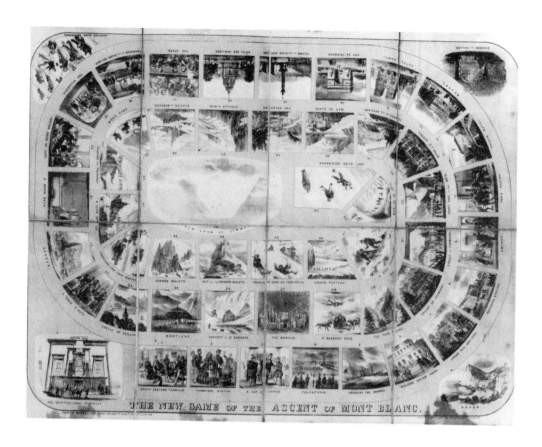

The New Game of the Ascent of Mont Blanc, by Albert Smith (*Alpine Club Collection, London*)

pairs of cloth trousers, two pairs of gaiters, two waistcoats, a shooting coat, and over all a blue woollen smock-frock. His sufferings commenced at the Mur de la Côte, where his friends passed him. He was supported by [the guides] Folliguet and the younger Couttet . . . a lethargy came over him, and a burning thirst which a mouthful of vinegar taken every now and then only partly assuaged. At half-past ten, about eight hours after leaving the *Grands Mulets*, they reached the summit. Atkins descended a little on the south side to obtain warmth, wrapped himself in a blanket and went fast asleep. Waking up in a few minutes he enjoyed a splendid view, but, like Dr Paccard, he lost his hat, and tied five handkerchiefs around his head. After remaining on the top a little more than an hour, they descended and arrived at the *Grands Mulets* at three in the afternoon . . . They arrived at Chamonix in the evening. Hedrengen's eyes were

greatly inflamed, Pidwel was horribly blistered, Atkins suffered much from weakness and was laid up for a week unable
to use his limbs, but shortly recovered and was able to
resume his studies. The Countess K . . . who thought he
was lost, attended a dinner given in his honour, and proposed his health, wishing that the same success might attend
his military career as had attended him in his ascent of Mont
Blanc. The excursion cost each of the three travellers twenty
pounds.[8]

Of all those who managed to scale the great mountain, however, Albert Smith must be the oddest. He was born the son of a
country surgeon, and in 1826, at the age of ten, was given a small
book, *The Peasants of Chamonix*, which gave a graphic account
of Dr Hamel's ill-fated expedition in 1820 when three guides were
lost in a crevasse. From then on he became obsessed with Mont
Blanc, and, while still a child, 'produced a small moving pano-
rama of the horrors pertaining to Mont Blanc'.

In 1838, while a medical student in Paris, he managed to travel
to Geneva with a fellow student, the journey taking seventy-eight
hours. They went on to Chamonix, where they inspected the
glaciers, before continuing their journey to Italy. Whymper tells
us, in *A Guide to Chamonix and the Range of Mont Blanc*:

> . . . Shortly after his return he thought he could make a
> grand lecture about the Alps. 'I copied,' he said 'all my
> pictures on a comparatively large scale – about three feet
> high – with such daring lights and shadows, and streaks of
> sunset, that I have since trembled at my temerity as I looked
> at them; and then, contriving some simple mechanism with a
> carpenter to make them roll on, I produced a lecture which
> in the town [Chertsey] was quite a 'hit'. . . . For two or three
> years, with my Alps in a box, I went round to various literary
> institutions. . . . I recall these first efforts of a show-man –
> for such they really were – with great pleasure. I recollect
> how my brother and I used to drive our four-wheeled chaise
> across the country, with Mont Blanc on the back seat.

Smith, it need scarcely be said, gave up all idea of medicine,
and in fact pursued a literary career, writing for *Punch*. Eventually, he returned to Chamonix. It was 1851, and by chance
W.E. Sackville-West, Mr Francis Phillips and Mr C.C. Floyd –
all young men from Oxford – decided to make the climb at the

same time. 'They were informed that a Mr Smith of London wished to accompany them. As they had no acquaintance with Smith they declined the honour, but finding out later that it was Mr Albert Smith, the well-known comic author, they introduced themselves, and proposed to make one party, to which he readily assented.'[9]

There follows an account of the ascent, for which the unfortunate Smith was not physically prepared. After the traditional stop for sleep at the Grands Mulets, they proceeded on their way.

. . . The route was of course perfectly easy, and it is difficult to comprehend Smith's assertion that 'Every step we took was gained from the chance of a horrible death'. Working up the Corridor, they made for the *Rochers Rouges* . . . The sun rose, but the north-east wind was bitterly cold, and Smith, who was chilled and dispirited, was nearly at the end of his resources. At the foot of the *Mur de la Côte* he sat down on the snow, told his guides he would go no further, and that they might leave him there if they pleased. The guides were accustomed to these ebullitions of temper at that elevation; they induced the jaded traveller to get his wandering wits in order, and the party plodded steadily on . . . An hour was occupied in getting to the top of the *Mur*, when Smith could hardly combat an irrepressible desire to sleep, but he was dragged on; his senses were not under control, and he reeled and staggered like a drunk man. His physical condition was the only excuse for his gross exaggeration in describing this well-known ice-slope.

'It is an all but perpendicular iceberg. You begin to ascend it obliquely, there is no thing below but a chasm in the ice, more frightful than anything yet passed. Should the foot slip or the baton give way there is no chance for life. You would glide like lightening from one frozen crag to another, and finally be dashed to pieces hundreds and hundreds of feet below, in the horrible depths of the glacier'.

As a matter of fact the *Mur de la Côte*, though one of the steepest bits of the journey, is perfectly safe, and the traveller, if he fell upon it, would be landed on soft snow at the bottom, the only drawback being that the climb so far must be made over again. It is plain that C.E. Mathews is shocked as much by Albert Smith's powers of exaggeration as by his pusillamity, failing to appreciate, no doubt, that a man with his sense of drama would not only instinctively

Drawing by Rodolphe Töpffer (from *Nouveaux Voyages en Zigzag*)

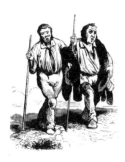

'embroider' the details of such a climb, but would also undergo mental suffering unknown to more down-to-earth mountaineers. One cannot help sympathising with C.E. Mathew's censure, however, as one continues to read Albert's description of the *Mur de la Côte*. 'Placed 14,000 feet above the level of the sea, [on a spot] terminating in an icy abyss so deep that the bottom is lost in obscurity, exposed, in a highly rarefied atmosphere, to a wind cold and violent beyond all conception, assailed with muscular power already taxed far beyond its strength, and nerves shaken by constantly increasing excitement and want of rest, with bloodshot eyes and a raging thirst, and a pulse leaping rather than beating; with all this, it may be imagined that the frightful *Mur de la Côte* calls for more than ordinary determination to mount it.' Mount it he did, though, thanks to the guides, who 'kept on dragging at the rope, steps were cut . . . Smith – sometimes falling on his hands and knees – was absolutely exhausted, but the tug of the rope was inexorable, and almost at his last gasp, he found that the ardent wish of years was gratified and that he was on the summit of Mont Blanc. He fell on the snow and was asleep in an instant, but after a few minutes' rest, he recovered, and the day being cloudless he was able to get some satisfaction from the Great Spectacle which was unfolded to his view.

'Nine months afterwards,' Whymper tells us, '[Albert Smith] produced at the Egyptian Hall, Piccadilly, an entertainment descriptive of the ascent, which "took the world by storm, and became the most popular exhibition of the kind ever known".' The effect was immediate. Whereas in the sixty-four years from 1786 to the end of 1850 there had been only fifty-seven ascents of Mont Blanc, in the six years 1852–7 there were sixty-four ascents. It is due to Albert Smith to say that his influence extended far beyond Chamonix and Mont Blanc. Many people date their first craving for the Alps from the time when they heard this able lecturer and genial showman.

Notes

1. *Voyage dans les Alpes*, Horace Benedict de Saussure, Volume IV, chapter II.
2. *A Guide to Chamonix and the Range of Mont Blanc*, Edward Whymper, John Murray, London, 1896.

3. From Note by Douglas W. Freshfield following the reprinted paper by Colonel Beaufoy, read to the Royal Society on 13 December, 1787, which is included in the *Alpine Journal* of 1915, Vol. 29. Douglas Freshfield wrote: 'The paper here reprinted is copied from the original MS, hidden in the archives of the Royal Society. It remained unprinted until 1817, when it appeared in the February number of the *Annals of Philosophy*.'
4. Printed for Gwendolyn Beaufoy, Basil Blackwell, Oxford, 1930.
5. Gwendolyn Beaufoy wrote: 'Margaretta, from her picture by Downman, must have been a very pretty young woman. She seems to have kept the family accounts from the day she eloped with Mark Beaufoy, and has left a most delightful account-book: *Leaves from a Beech Tree*.
6. *A Guide to Chamonix and the Range of Mont Blanc*, Edward Whymper, John Murray, 1896.
7. *The Annals of Mont Blanc*, C.E. Mathews, T. Fisher-Unwin, 1898.
8. 'Ascent to the Summit of Mont Blanc on the 22 and 23 August, 1837', Not published, Calkin and Budd, London, 1838.
9. *The Annals of Mont Blanc*, C.E. Mathews, T. Fisher Unwin, 1890.

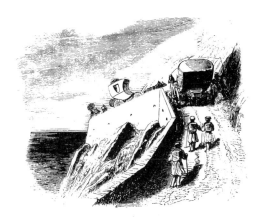

EPILOGUE

As I write this, a plane from London is due to touch down at Geneva's airport. Out of it will spill hopeful skiers, some on their way to Chamonix perhaps. Possibly, too, there may be a young Hentsch or Pictet, home from a six months' stint in London, and perhaps an English expert from the United Nations' Narcotics Board. The airport is large and sophisticated, and will of course be bristling with international security precautions. What a far cry this from Dejean's *calèches*, waiting to convey English visitors halfway across Europe to the Hôtel d'Angleterre! And yet, the travellers we have lived with in these pages have not totally vanished from the Old Geneva scene. They have been absorbed into the very fabric of the city. Their manuscripts, paintings, and accounts of mountain exploits are in state archives, private collections and libraries. Above all, though, they are alive in the collective memory of the Genevese. You feel this, when you live in Geneva as their compatriot, in the late twentieth century.

October, 1988
Hampshire